Transforming Nursing Data Into Quality Care:

Profiles of Quality Improvement in U.S. Healthcare Facilities

Isis Montalvo, RN, MS, MBA

Nancy Dunton, PhD

Editors

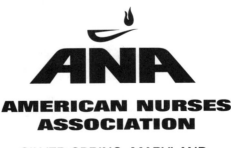

AMERICAN NURSES ASSOCIATION

SILVER SPRING, MARYLAND

2007

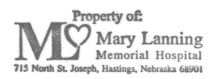

Library of Congress Cataloging-in-Publication data

Transforming nursing data into quality care : profiles of quality improvement in U.S. healthcare facilities/ Isis Montalvo and Nancy Dunton, editors.

    p. ; cm.

    Includes bibliographical references and index.

    ISBN-13: 978-1-55810-249-1 (pbk.)

    ISBN-10: 1-55810-249-3 (pbk.)

    1. Nursing–United States–Quality control. 2. Hospitals–United States–Quality control. I. Montalvo, Isis. II. Dunton, Nancy. III. American Nurses Association.

    [DNLM: 1. Nursing Process–United States. 2. Quality Indicators, Health Care–United States. 3. Health Facilities–United States. 4. Quality Assurance, Health Care–standards–United States. WY 100 T772 2007]

RT85.5.T73 2007

610.73068–dc222007001440

Published by Nursesbooks.org
The Publishing Program of ANA

American Nurses Association
8515 Georgia Avenue, Suite 400
Silver Spring, MD 20910-3492
1-800-274-4ANA
http://www.nursesbooks.org/

ANA is the only full-service professional organization representing the nation's 2.9 million Registered Nurses through its 54 constituent member associations. The ANA advances the nursing profession by fostering high standards of nursing practice, promoting the economic and general welfare of nurses in the workplace, projecting a positive and realistic view of nursing, and lobbying the Congress and regulatory agencies on healthcare issues affecting nurses and the public.

Design and composition: Laura Johnson/LJ Design, *Editing:* Bill Robinson, Grammarians, Inc., *Project assistance:* Mellen Candage, Grammarians, Inc., Alexandria, VA.
Printing: McArdle Printing, Upper Marlboro, MD.

ISBN-13: 978-1-55810-249-1   ISBN-10: 1-55810-249-3   SAN: 851-3481
07NDNQ   2.5M   01/07
First printing: January 2007

Contents

About the Editors

Isis Montalvo, RN, MS, MBA
Manager, Nursing Practice & Policy
American Nurses Association

Isis Montalvo is Manager, Nursing Practice and Policy, and is primarily responsible for providing oversight to the National Database of Nursing Quality Indicators (NDNQI®). She has over 19 years experience in multiple areas of critical care clinical practice and management in a large acute care setting. She has held clinical education, leadership, management, and performance improvement positions throughout her career. In addition to her dual Master's from the University of Maryland System, she is a Critical Care Registered Nurse (CCRN) Alumnus. Ms. Montalvo is a member of the American Association of Critical Care Nurses, the Greater Washington Society of Association Executives, Phi Kappa Phi and Sigma Theta Tau Honor Societies.

Nancy Dunton, PhD
Director, National Database of
Nursing Quality Indicators

Nancy Dunton is a multi-talented researcher who brings many abilities to the National Database of Nursing Quality Indicators (NDNQI). She has been the director of NDNQI since its inception in 1998, guiding its growth development over the last eight years. Dr. Dunton has made numerous presentations on NDNQI to nurses across the United States and internationally. She has more than 25 years of experience in helping organizations use outcome indicators in decision making. Dr. Dunton is a Research Associate Professor in the University of Kansas Medical Center's School of Nursing, with a joint appointment in the Department of Health Policy and Management. She has been the principal investigator on more than 20 health and social services research projects and has served on committees for National Quality Forum, the Agency for Healthcare Quality and Research, and the Committee on National Statistics of the National Academy of Sciences. Dr. Dunton received her PhD in Sociology from the University of Wisconsin–Madison.

Acknowledgements

The editors would like to thank the staff nurses who make the daily difference in patient outcomes, the profile authors for their generosity in sharing their experiences so others might benefit and the following people for their time, commitment and involvement on various levels: Eric Wurzbacher, Mary Jean Schumann RN, MSN, MBA, CPNP, Pam Hagan, MSN, RN, Peggy Miller MS, RN, Belinda Pierson, MA, Angela Christopher, BSN, RN, Jan Davidson, MSN, ARNP, Byron Gajewski, PhD and Susan Klaus, PhD, RN.

INTRODUCTION: Achieving Sustained Healthcare Improvements Through the Use of Nursing Quality Indicators

History of NDNQI

The word nursing has long been synonymous with caring, compassion, healing, and trust. Nurses frequently top the list as the most trusted and ethical professionals, according to public opinion polls (Gallup 2006). Nursing's role in patient safety, improving practice, and patient outcomes has its roots in Florence Nightingale's work and is reflected in the American Nurses Association's (ANA) foundational documents.

Code of Ethics for Nurses with Interpretive Statements (ANA 2001) identifies that: "The nurse promotes, advocates for, and strives to protect the health, safety, and rights of the patient." This particular provision recognizes the nursing profession's responsibility to implement and maintain standards of professional practice, which includes planning, establishing, implementing, and evaluating quality improvement initiatives.

In *Nursing's Scope and Standards of Practice"* (ANA 2004), Standard 7 states: "The registered nurse systematically enhances the quality and effectiveness of nursing practice." Measurement criteria vary from identifying what factors or indicators need to be monitored, to using the results to change practice and improve healthcare systems.

The ANA has been in the forefront of health quality indicator development. In 1994, as part of ANA's Patient Safety and Quality Initiative, it supported a project to evaluate the linkages between nurse staffing and patient outcomes. Ten "nursing-sensitive indicators" were defined and adopted by ANA based on a review of the published evidence.

Nursing sensitive indicators reflect (a) characteristics of the nursing workforce, (b) nursing processes, or (c) patient outcomes that vary according to the characteristics or processes of nursing. Examples of nursing characteristics include measures of the supply of nursing, such as total nursing hours per patient day, or nursing skill, such as the percent of nursing hours supplied by RNs. Examples of nursing processes include risk assessment and protocol implementation. Examples of nursing-sensitive outcomes include fall rates which are related to nursing hours, and hospital-acquired pressure ulcer rates which are related to skill mix.

Subsequently, ANA supported seven state nurses associations, from across all regions of the United States, to conduct pilot studies to test the feasibility of collecting and reporting the indicators. In 1998, based on four years of development work, ANA established the National Database of Nursing Quality Indicators

(NDNQI®), which is administered by the University of Kansas Medical Center under contract to ANA. Participation in NDNQI has grown from the original 30 hospitals in the state pilot projects to over 1,000 facilities today. There is great diversity among participating facilities. NDNQI facilities are located in all 50 states and the District of Columbia. They include academic medical centers, other teaching facilities, and non-teaching facilities. They are located in metropolitan areas and rural communities, and include for profit, nonprofit, and government facilities. New facilities join the national database on an ongoing basis.

Nursing's Role in Quality

Nursing's role in quality and improving patient outcomes has its origin with Florence Nightingale, who identified fresh air, light, warmth, cleanliness, and efficient drainage as good for patients (Nightingale 1860). These were environmental and practice recommendations for nursing that could improve patient's health outcomes. Nightingale also utilized statistical methods to compare the mortality of patients based on the healthcare environment. She presented data, diagrammed causes of mortality, and calculated mortality rates in a report to England's Royal Commission. She analyzed data on surgical outcomes and provided data on the mortality and morbidity of children. She created statistical forms and made many other contributions. Nightingale became the first female inducted into the London Statistical Society/Royal Statistical Society (Dossey 2005).

Development of Quality Improvement Models

The field of quality statistical control measurement accelerated in the early 1920s with the advancement of quality control methods in manufacturing. Theorists such as Joseph Juran, W. Edwards Deming, and A. Feigenbaum added to the quality management body of knowledge and made significant contributions to quality management theory. The works of Walter A. Shewhart, H.F. Dodge, H.G. Romig, K. Ishikawa, G. Taguchi, and others are widely recognized as contributing to the development of quality improvement tools. The current spectrum of quality improvement approaches is very broad, ranging from quality control to quality improvement, continuous quality improvement, Total Quality Management (TQM), Six Sigma, and the International Standardization Organization (ISO) Quality Management System.

Most of these approaches urge organizations to set goals, develop measures of goal achievement, collect and review data, make improvements, and then check subsequent data to see if the improvements had the desired results.

NDNQI's Approach to Collecting Data

NDNQI's approach to collecting data for quality improvement is based on Avedis Donabedian's conceptual framework (Donabedian 1966, 1980, 1982), which holds that the structure of care affects the processes of care and that both, in turn, affect the outcomes of care. Therefore, NDNQI collects data on nursing *structure, process,* and *outcome* indicators, which provide a comprehensive approach to evaluating quality.

An example of this three-part approach, when addressing patient falls in a facility, is the use of: total nursing hours per patient day as a structure indicator; the percent of patients assessed for fall risk as a process indicator; and the number of patients who fell per 1,000 patient days as an outcome indicator. Together, these indicators provide an overall framework to evaluate and subsequently improve quality.

Measurement is an important step to improve quality. "Who, What, Why, When and How" are important questions that need to be answered in order to outline an improvement process. NDNQI provides the foundational framework and information for the bedside

Transforming Nursing Data Into Quality Care:
Profiles of Quality Improvement in U.S. Healthcare Facilities

nurse, the nurse manager, the nurse educator, the nurse researcher, the clinical nurse specialist (CNS), and the nurse executive to evaluate and answer these questions and, subsequently, to improve the nursing process.

NDNQI provides the tools necessary to improve patient care at the facility level, the unit level, and for individual nurses as well. NDNQI provides each nurse the opportunity to review the evidence, evaluate their practice, and determine what improvements can be made. This is important to the healthcare system, especially since healthcare systems have increasingly become concerned with patient safety. Several of the Institute of Medicine's (IOM) reports (IOM 1999, 2001, 2005) highlight key areas of concern for patient safety, areas needed for improvement, and the actions required to accelerate improvements. NDNQI provides necessary information to the nurse and the healthcare facility to assist in improving patient safety.

NDNQI's Development of Nursing-sensitive Indicators

NDNQI's work in the development of nursing-sensitive indicators not only supports nursing (to affect and improve patient safety), but also improve healthcare quality. The development of reliable and valid nursing-sensitive indicators is a multi-step process that includes:

- Reviewing scientific literature for: (a) evidence that some aspect of nursing care has an effect on a patient outcome; (b) specific definitions of the indicators; and (c) evidence that the indicators can be validly and reliably measured,

- Collecting information from researchers in the field on threats to reliability and validity,

- Conducting expert review of draft indicator definitions, data collection guidelines, and data collection forms,

- Distributing revised definitions, guidelines, and forms to clinical experts for comments on face validity and feasibility of reliable data collection,

- Incorporating clinical expert feedback and developing revised versions of definitions, guidelines, and forms,

- Conducting a pilot study using the draft data collection materials and reviewing data and interviewing hospital study coordinators to identify additional threats to reliability and validity,

- Finalizing definitions, data collection guidelines, and forms, and

- Training database participants in standardized data collection practices.

Out of ANA's 10 original nursing-sensitive indicators, six have been fully tested and developed (Appendix A).[1] Four of the NDNQI indicators (total nursing hours per patient day, skill mix, fall rates, and injury fall rates) have been accepted by the National Quality Forum (NQF) as national consensus measures. NQF was established by the U.S. Congress as the standards development body for healthcare quality, with the intent of providing a national strategy for healthcare quality and reporting to facilitate system-wide quality improvement (NQF 2004). NQF adopted a total of 15 nursing-sensitive indicators (NQF NS-15) in 2004 (Appendix B). NQF has many other categories of indicators; however, the NQF NS-15 are the only nursing-sensitive indicators set by NQF at this time. NDNQI continues to add to its database NQF-endorsed measures. Within the last year, two additional NQF measures were made available to participating facilities (practice environment scale and prevalence of restraint use) and, currently, four NQF indicators are being prepared for deployment through NDNQI (voluntary nurse turnover, urinary catheter-associated urinary tract infections, ventilator-associated pneumonias, and central line-associated blood stream infections).

---

1. The four patient satisfaction indicators were never developed, because differences in questionnaire and data collection procedures across hospitals precluded the collection of standardized information.

Uses for Healthcare Quality Indicators

Healthcare consumers, regulators, and providers increasingly are engaged in initiatives to make healthcare quality information transparent to the consumer. This new use for quality indicators is generating discussion as to whether indicators should be adjusted for hospital differences in patient acuity before being made public. Some maintain that hospitals with more acutely ill patients will look worse on quality measures because of their patient populations, rather than due to the quality of care they provide. Others argue that the intensity of nursing services reported should be increased to match patient acuity and that the indicators should not be adjusted. At the time of this publication, the debate was ongoing.

Another new use for healthcare quality indicators is "pay for performance" (P4P), under which hospitals that achieve high quality of care in an efficient manner are rewarded by insurance companies and government with higher reimbursement rates. Recently, the Centers for Medicaid and Medicare Services (CMS) has started using the term "Value Based Purchasing" (VBP). To date, nursing quality indicators have not been incorporated in many of these programs.

Future of NDNQI

NDNQI is never in a static state and is frequently modified as the database has its own quality improvement process. New indicators are developed and added yearly, while old indicators and data collection tools are modified and upgraded in accordance with new evidence from clinical practice. This process is designed to further enhance reliability and validity based on internal studies, and to reduce the data collection burden on hospitals. NDNQI engages in multiple avenues for training facilities' personnel in standardized data collection and for providing technical assistance. Over the years, NDNQI has evolved from one-time, telephone-based training, to a system that includes an on-line tutorial, newsletters, quarterly teleconferences, and annual conferences. New report designs and delivery systems are integrated into operations on an ongoing basis. Input from hospitals on how they use the reports and what new features they would like is important to NDNQI.

NDNQI Profiles

This monograph provides a perspective from a diverse selection of hospitals throughout the United States on their experience with NDNQI, their efforts to improve patient outcomes, and their success stories. NDNQI analyzed several years of data to identify facilities that had sustained improvement in one or more of the nursing-sensitive indicators. Those facilities were asked to share their quality improvement process in this volume—what worked, what didn't work, how they achieved success, who was involved, and what they learned.

These hospitals have transformed NDNQI nursing data into sustained improvements in quality outcomes. They have generously shared their experiences in the following chapters so that others might learn and improve their own practices. It is their experiences, their stories, in their own words.

We think Florence Nightingale would be very proud of NDNQI and the work that these nurses, their predecessors, successors, and the nursing community have done to continuously improve nursing practice, patient safety, and patient outcomes.

Isis Montalvo, RN, MS, MBA
Manager, Division of Practice and Policy
American Nurses Association

Nancy Dunton, PhD
Director, National Database of Nursing
    Quality Indicators
Research Associate Professor, University of
    Kansas Medical Center School of Nursing;
    Department of Health Policy and Management

References

American Nurses Association. *Code of ethics for nurses with interpretive statements.* Silver Spring, MD: Nursesbooks.org; 2001.

American Nurses Association. *Nursing: Scope and standards of practice.* Silver Spring, MD.: Nursesbooks.org; 2004.

Donabedian A. Evaluating the quality of medical care. *Milbank Memorial Fund Quarterly* 1966; 44:166–206. (On-line access at www.PubMed.gov under PMID: 5338568.)

Donabedian A. *Explorations in quality assessment and monitoring. Vol. I. The definition of quality and approaches to its assessment.* Ann Arbor: Health Administration Press; 1980.

Donabedian A. *Explorations in quality assessment and monitoring. Vol. II.* The criteria and standards of quality. Ann Arbor: Health Administration Press; 1982.

Dossey BM, Selanders LC, Beck D-M, Attewell A. *Florence Nightingale today: Healing, leadership, global action.* Silver Spring, MD: Nursesbooks.org; 2005.

The Gallup Poll.© Nurses top list of most honest and ethical professions. The Gallup Organization: Princeton, NJ; December 14, 2006. (On-line access at http://www.galluppoll.com/. Poll numbers available online at http://www.usatoday.com/news/polls/tables/live/2006-12-11-ethics.htm)

Institute of Medicine. *To err is human: Building a safer health system.* Washington, DC: National Academies Press; 1999. (On-line access at http://www.iom.edu/CMS/8089/5575.aspx)

Institute of Medicine. *Crossing the quality chasm.* Washington, DC: National Academies Press; 2001. (On-line access at http://www.iom.edu/CMS/8089/5432.aspx)

Institute of Medicine. *Performance measurement: Accelerating improvement.* Washington, DC: National Academies Press; 2005. (On-line access at http://www.iom.edu/?id=34827)

Nightingale F. *Notes on nursing: What it is, and what it is not.* London: Harrison and Sons; 1860.

National Quality Forum. *National voluntary consensus standards for nursing-sensitive care: An initial performance measure set.* Washington, DC: NQF; 2004. (Executive summary available on-line at http://www.qualityforum.org/pdf/reports/nsc.pdf)

Physical/Sexual Assaults

Defined:

Assaults are defined by the NDNQI® as unwanted **physical** contact by a patient **whether or not** there is intent to harm. Some patients may be confused or otherwise not understand a situation and strike out. This type of unintentional assault is included in the definition. *The NDNQI definition of assault **does not** include verbal threats or nonverbal intimidation.*

Physical assaults involve the use of force and include pushing, scratching, punching, kicking, slapping, biting, spitting, intentional body fluid spray, and thrown objects that hit another person. Sexual assaults are unwanted sexual contacts and include rape, attempted rape, fondling, and forced kissing.

A physical or sexual assault may or may not result in injury.

The assault can be directed at staff members, students, other patients, or visitors. **Do not** include self-inflicted harm by the patient.

The assault must be performed by a patient. **Exclude** assaultive behaviors demonstrated by:

- Visitors
- Students
- Staff members
- Patients on units not eligible for reporting
- Patients on units eligible for reporting, but **not on the unit** at time of the assaultive behavior (e.g., patient assaultive episode occurred in a recreational therapy activity held off the unit)

Formula:

(Number of Assaults X 1000)/Total Number of Patient Days

NDNQI Assault Data on Unit Dashboards Results in Improved Management of Aggressive Behavior

Kathy Szumanski, MSN, RN, CNA-BC
Director, Clinical Excellence and Professional Development
Kathy.Szumanski@advocatehealth.com

Advocate Lutheran General Hospital—Park Ridge, Illinois

Editors' pick:

INSIGHTS & IDEAS FROM THIS FACILITY

Ensured oversight for consistent data across units, integrated program into daily operations, and involved all staff.

Facility Summary

Facility	Advocate Lutheran General Hospital—Park Ridge, Illinois **www.Advocatehealth.com**
Facility setting	Suburban, full-service hospital
Teaching status	Teaching hospital
Ownership	Nonprofit
Community demographics	Northwestern Cook County, Illinois presents diverse communities, with 15 languages spoken in an area with population expansion.
Number of hospital beds	617
Indicators used	All available NDNQI indicators
System or unit improved	Unit improvement—Mental health
Indicators improved	Assault management
QI document	Quarterly individual unit dashboard
NDNQI participant	2003–present
Magnet™ status	Magnet designation August 2005

UNIT PROFILE

Unit size and type	52-bed mental health unit
Unit RN staff profile	Average RN years on unit: 10.2 RN national board certification 25%
Skill mix of RNs, other personnel	36.8 FTE RNs, 21.8 FTE mental health workers, 9 FTE nursing care technicians, 5.5 FTE secretaries
Organizational structure of unit	One clinical manager (Doctorally-prepared) Three assistant clinical managers (BSN-prepared) One clinical educator (MSN-prepared)

Transforming Nursing Data Into Quality Care:
Profiles of Quality Improvement in U.S. Healthcare Facilities

NDNQI Assault Data on Unit Dashboards Results in Improved Management of Aggressive Behavior

Kathy Szumanski, MSN, RN, CNA-BC
Director, Clinical Excellence and Professional Development
Kathy.Szumanski@advocatehealth.com

Introductory Summary:
Advocate Lutheran General and Assaults

Nursing in the hospital clinical arena, as practiced today, may present as a complex maze of practice challenges, mandatory elements of care, expanding electronic documentation modalities, and frequent change. Process improvement activities in this kind of turbulence require thoughtful focus and a steady hand to produce meaningful results. A quality focus in the mental health units of Advocate Lutheran General Hospital (ALGH) has involved a study of assaultive behavior and the development of an improvement program that targets the identification and management of aggressive or agitated behavior in that setting. By participating in the National Database for Nursing Quality Indicators (NDNQI) database on assaultive behavior, the mental health units have been able to quantify, trend, and analyze their efforts.

Introductory Summary:
Facility at a Glance

Advocate Lutheran General Hospital is a 617-bed tertiary care teaching hospital with Level 1 Trauma designation that is located in northwest Cook County just outside the Chicago Metropolitan area. ALGH is also home to the ALGH Children's Hospital, a comprehensive provider of children's services in the state. The pediatric division supports a Level 3 Neonatal Intensive Care Unit. ALGH has been recognized as a leader in advanced treatment capabilities in cardiology, cancer care, critical care neurology, orthopedics, women's health, and trauma care. Solucient has named the hospital as one of the nation's top 100 hospitals for the last 10 years. In August 2005, ALGH was also awarded Magnet designation. There are over 1,000 physicians on staff and approximately 1,200 nurses practice at ALGH. Undergraduate, graduate, and medical students from 18 academic institutions send students to ALGH for clinical rotations.

Advocate Lutheran General Hospital is one of eight hospitals in the Oakbrook Illinois-based Advocate Health Care System that is the largest fully integrated nonprofit health care delivery system in Illinois. ALGH is a full-service hospital and cares for patients in all age ranges. The inpatient and outpatient scope includes all levels of complexity from ambulatory care to critical care. A full continuum of care is provided.

A market assessment of the suburban geographic ring of ALGH shows a current racial mix that is: 75.8% white, 8.4% Hispanic, 11.6% Asian, 2.6% black, and a multiracial mix of 1.5% which includes Native Ameri-

Physical/Sexual Assaults:
NDNQI Assault Data on Unit Dashboards Results in Improved Management of Aggressive Behavior

11

cans. Of this racial mix, the age distribution shows 29.4% in the 45-66 age group and 33.8% in the 18-44 age group.

The overall population growth in this market exceeds the national rates in both the primary service area and the secondary service area. There are 15 different languages spoken by patients who are admitted to ALGH.

Nurses who practice at ALGH are committed to achieving the best patient outcomes by providing high-quality patient care. ALGH has focused attention on nursing quality initiatives at all levels of care. Standards of practice are the frame of reference for nursing care and the continuous quality improvement process is used to identify high-risk concerns or aspects of care where opportunities for improvement exist.

The nursing governance model provides the venue in which input from practicing nurses is gathered for the development and monitoring of quality plans. Each unit or department has a staff nurse as a "quality anchor" who is identified as a champion for process improvement. Participation in the NDNQI database has created a strong opportunity to integrate quality into ALGH nursing care and has solidified the opportunity for the quality anchor to incorporate and interpret quality results for all members of the unit. The opportunity to have comparative national benchmarks and trends for quality indicators through participation in the NDNQI has been beneficial to the mental health units at ALGH.

The management teams of the behavioral health areas consist of a clinical manager who is a doctorally prepared registered nurse certified in mental health and three assistant clinical managers who have baccalaureate degrees. There are 36.8 full-time equivalent (FTEs) RNs who provide direct patient care. Supplementing the professional nursing staff are 21.8 FTE mental health workers, 9 FTE nursing care technicians, and 5.5 FTE secretaries. Although the direct caregivers are assigned to one of the three clinical

units, they are also cross-trained and able to float among the three units. The average number of years experience for the nurse caregivers is 10.2 and 25% of the nurses have national board certification. A master's prepared clinical educator provides educational support for the entire team.

NDNQI Startup Considerations

ALGH has participated in NDNQI since 2003 to allow comparative analysis in a national database, with a set of nurse-sensitive quality indicators receiving focused attention. There are many risk factors for aggressive behavior in a mental health setting that occur not only due to the psychiatric components of illness but also due to the limited setting and environmental confinement needed for treatments. Interventions aimed at establishing control and assuring safety must be initiated when certain triggers are recognized.

The quality team on these units determined that an improvement initiative related to managing aggression would assist them to assure that a milieu for optimal treatment could be maintained. They determined the need to study the rates, frequency, and types of physical/sexual assault incidences, and that it would be desirable to explore the relationship between assaultive episodes and nursing experience, staffing, and training. While enthusiastic about the opportunity to see how the ALGH setting compared to others, the staff struggled at first with the definitions of the desired indicators. Discussion groups, with case study presentations, helped pave the way for enthusiastic buy-in for the quality initiative.

Quality Measurement and Reporting

Each of the behavioral health units has designed a quality dashboard that contains its key quality indicators with goals, national benchmarks where appropriate, and trends over time to mark their progress. A physical/sexual assault indicator is included on the mental

FIGURE 1.

Recording Quality Indicator Data—an ALGH Quality Dashboard

Advocate Lutheran General Hospital
Unit Quality Dashboard
2006

n/a = not applicable
n.d. = no data
NDNQI MEAN = National Comparative Information – Bed Size >= 500

5 Center – LOS	Jan	Feb	Mar	Apr	May	Jun	Jul	Aug	Sept	Oct	Nov	Dec
Average Unit LOS												
National Mean LOS (HCFA)												
Actual to National Mean Comparison (variance)												

Indicator

5 Center - Physical/Sexual Assault	Goal		Q1			Q2			Q3			Q4
Injury Assault Rates	0.00											
Total Assault Rates												

Goal

Results

Patient Charac.
	Goal
Median Age	
% Male	
% Involuntary Admission	

Characteristics of Injury Assaults
Median Time Since Admission (Days)
% Within 24 Hours of Admission
% Repeat Assaults
Mean Number Assault Victims
% Nurse Victims

Job Classifications of Injured Persons (May not = 100% due to undocumented classification not reported)
RN
LPN
UAP/MHT
Social Worker, etc.
Other HC Provider
Security
Other Patient
Visitor
Any Other Person

Injury Level Most Severely Injured Person
Non Nurse
Minor
Moderate
Major
Nurse
Minor
Moderate
Major

Charac. of Nurse Victims
Years Psych Nursing Experience – Mean
% w/ Assault Management Training

Post Assault Intervention (Percentages will sum to >100, as multiple interventions are used)
None
Calmly Talk to Patient
Instruct: Leave Area
Escort Patient from Area
1:1 Observation
Called Security
Restrained
Seclusion
Other

5 Center- Physical/Sexual Assault (cont.)	Goal		Q1			Q2			Q3			Q4

Restraint Types/Duration/Secl. Median % Use Restr. Type Dur.
Holds
Pharmacological
Devices
Restraint Devices (Hours)
Seclusion (Hours)

Skill Mix	Goal	NDNQI MEAN	Q1	NDNQI MEAN	Q2	NDNQI MEAN	Q3	NDNQI MEAN	Q4
Total Nursing Hrs per Patient Day	> Mean								
RN Hrs per Patient Day	> Mean								
% of Total Nursing Hours Supplied by RNs – **Psych**	> Mean								
% of Total Nursing Hours Supplied by LPNs/LVNs – **Psych**									
% of Total Nursing Hours Supplied by UAPs – **Psych**	@ Mean								
% of Total Nursing Hours Supplied by Agency Staff – **Psych**	< Mean								

Inpatient Behavioral Health – Advocate Experience	BL	Goal	Jan	Feb	Mar	Apr	May	Jun	Jul	Aug	Sept	Oct	Nov	Dec
Overall Question – Percent Very Good														
Total # of Responses														

5 Center – Chart Audits	Goal	Jan	Feb	Mar	Apr	May	Jun	Jul	Aug	Sept	Oct	Nov	Dec
Presence of Documentation of Medication Education Present in Chart													
Telephone orders are Read Back and Signed by Nurse													
History and Physical Within 24 hours													
No Use of Unapproved Abbreviations, Acronyms, or Symbols													
Treatment Plan Updated													

This document was prepared for ALGH's internal performance improvement and ,as such, is strictly confidential and is not admissible as evidence in any action of any kind in any court of law pursuant to the Illinois Medical Studies Act.

health dashboards used in the units at ALGH (Figure 1). NDNQI defines assault as "unwanted contact with another person with intent to harm." The contact does not need to result in injury. Sexual assaults are "unwanted sexual contacts and include rape, attempted rape, fondling, forced kissing, and exposure."

The quality specialist populates the dashboard on an ongoing basis, and a completed dashboard is released to the units at quarterly intervals. At a unit nursing governance meeting, the staff nurse who is the "quality anchor" presents the unit results and there is a dialogue on problem solving for areas of challenge, a discussion of shared accountability, and the opportunity to highlight accomplishments of the team. The management team assists with the presentation and interpretation, if necessary.

The assigned quality specialist may also be invited to participate. At least four times a year, the unit presents a quality showcase for the nursing executive team representatives to communicate both successes and challenges. This is an excellent opportunity to foster dialogue between direct caregivers and senior leadership on a regular basis.

If the quality results are not within 10% of the predetermined goal, then an action plan is prepared by the unit to address areas of concerns. This action plan is submitted to the Quality Management Committee as part of the nursing report.

A unit dashboard can be amended to include staffing data to monitor for relationships between staffing levels and quality outcomes. Patient satisfaction results are usually added to unit dashboards so that the direct care team can see how their patients perceive their care delivery.

Clinical teams have a partnership with a quality specialist in the Quality Management Department in order to use their expertise in the creation of quality indicator statements that are clear, measurable, accepted, and for which it is possible to track results for specific settings. The Director of Clinical Excellence and Nursing Professional Development has oversight responsibility for the nursing quality program.

The application of evidence-based practice is a strategic priority in nursing. Its development and application is a goal of the Advance Practice Nursing Council, which receives guidance and support from the director of Nursing Research, Education, and Development. The integration of nursing research findings into clinical practice is a program that is refined as the ALGH nursing research program grows.

Currently, a total of 19 units submit quality data to the NDNQI. Three of these units provide care for patients requiring behavioral health services and all have an active quality program in place. The adult behavioral health unit is a 26-bed locked adult psychiatric unit that provides intensive psychiatric treatment to patients who have a variety of psychiatric and/or addiction disorders and need acute, intensive inpatient treatment. Patients on this unit may have dual diagnoses of an acute psychiatric disorder and addictions. There are some patients who present with secondary conditions such as developmental disorders, neurological disorders, delirium, and sensory deficits. Although patients with concurrent unstable medical conditions are not admitted, many will have subacute chronic medical problems.

A second behavioral health unit is a 14-bed geriatric-psychiatric unit that provides treatment to older adult patients (age 60+) who have a variety of psychiatric disorders and need acute, intensive inpatient treatment. Patients are admitted because of their inability to function as a result of a primary psychiatric diagnosis. Underlying conditions, such as dementia, neurological and sensory deficits, may also be present. Most patients have subacute chronic medical conditions that may require stabilization during their stay. The third behavioral health unit is a 12-bed child/adolescent psychiatric unit that provides care for patients who need crisis intervention, cognitive/behavioral therapy, coping skill management, medication stabilization, and reality orientation.

Quality Improvement: Using the Assault Indicator

During the development of the process improvement program on the mental health units, the team noted that the data related to assaults were variable, with the geriatric unit identifying many more incidents of assault than the more acute adult unit. When the units participated in the NDNQI's pilot study, it was found that each unit was working from a different set of definitions and counting frequency in different ways. These factors prompted the team to discard the ALGH data collection as it was designed and to study the phenomenon of assaults, mechanisms to de-escalate it, and begin an aggressive educational program.

The behavioral health units' commitment to excellence in care delivery involved the development of a program that was designed to manage aggressive patients as part of their ongoing sustained quality achievement, which was augmented by their experience in the NDNQI pilot study.

During the course of treatment in an inpatient behavioral health setting, aggressive or agitated behavior can develop. The potential for assault is very real and early intervention with escalating behavior can restore safety to the environment and control for the patient.

The multidisciplinary quality team was committed to avoiding repeated episodes of restraint and seclusion for patients and turned their attention to assessment of agitated behavior, early intervention, and rapid de-escalation as needed. By requiring all members of the team to participate in de-escalation training, cohesion and similarity of management of violent prevention was established.

The program moved through a series of specific phases:

- Define goals for the process improvement initiative.

- Review evidence-based practice on handling aggressive behavior.

- Develop an intervention program model.

- Identify metrics that would provide a measure of success.

- Educate members of the team.

- Monitor metrics of program success.

- Integrate the program into orientation and competency evaluation.

The toolkit that was developed as part of the management for aggressive patients included an aggressive patient management protocol, organizational policies on restraints and seclusion, procedures on the use of restraints in behavioral health, standing orders for behavioral control, an assault log and worksheet, a competency program with written examination, and the physical skills needed to restore control in a crisis.

The effort made in the design of a quality improvement program in the mental health setting has demonstrated good results. Over the past 18 months, the quality trends on assault rates were posted that are shown in Figure 2.

The quarterly quality data are reported and discussed at unit quality meetings and the team was been pleased with the degree of control that has been established and the improvement in overall unit safety. Assault rates from aggressive behavior have been reduced. A question that is frequently asked is: How much did this process improvement effort cost? There was no additional cost involved in the planning of the quality program because the opportunities for staff time existed with the nursing governance model that is in place in the organiza-

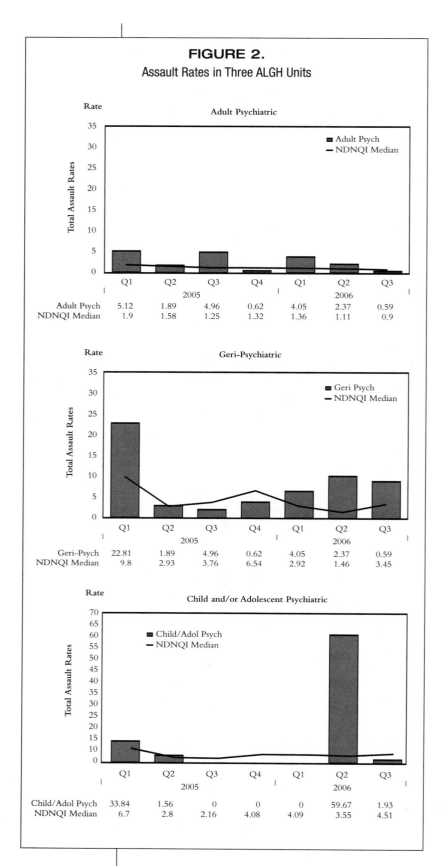

FIGURE 2.
Assault Rates in Three ALGH Units

Adult Psychiatric

Rate

Total Assault Rates

■ Adult Psych
— NDNQI Median

	Q1	Q2	Q3	Q4	Q1	Q2	Q3
	2005				2006		
Adult Psych	5.12	1.89	4.96	0.62	4.05	2.37	0.59
NDNQI Median	1.9	1.58	1.25	1.32	1.36	1.11	0.9

Geri-Psychiatric

Rate

Total Assault Rates

■ Geri Psych
— NDNQI Median

	Q1	Q2	Q3	Q4	Q1	Q2	Q3
	2005				2006		
Geri-Psych	22.81	1.89	4.96	0.62	4.05	2.37	0.59
NDNQI Median	9.8	2.93	3.76	6.54	2.92	1.46	3.45

Child and/or Adolescent Psychiatric

Rate

Total Assault Rates

■ Child/Adol Psych
— NDNQI Median

	Q1	Q2	Q3	Q4	Q1	Q2	Q3
	2005				2006		
Child/Adol Psych	33.84	1.56	0	0	0	59.67	1.93
NDNQI Median	6.7	2.8	2.16	4.08	4.09	3.55	4.51

tion. Approximately 568 hours of educational time, a one-time expense, was established for the de-escalation education program. The clinical educator assigned to the mental health area will be able to sustain this training effort within her budgeted educational responsibilities.

The opportunity to benchmark in the NDNQI database in behavioral health has allowed the comparison of similar work processes and outcomes across organizations. Learning from leading organizations in this way can solidify quality efforts and create the potential for scientific study through nursing research.

Lessons Learned

These highlights of the ALGH experience would prove helpful to any similar facility in its quality improvement efforts.

• Start small and keep it simple. In selecting meaningful indicators, start with a review of the existing evidence.

• Design a reporting template or unit dashboard to capture data related to specific quality indicators.

• Involve staff at every level of program development to assure long-term change.

• Integrate program elements into daily operations.

• Establish a data collection process and data flow reporting structure.

• Prepare quarterly reports and monitor trends.

• Take action when needed to correct variances.

• Celebrate successes and review barriers as a team.

While assaultive behavior will probably always be a part of the care on inpatient behavioral health units, establishing a quality management program focused on this indicator will bring a better level of care and more staff satisfaction with the work environment.

Conclusions and Implications

Nursing quality programs take time to grow and patience and dedication to improvement are essential in any initiative. Our participation in the NDNQI has helped us develop a strong focus on quality in our mental health units and to analyze data thoughtfully. Quality improvement is a dynamic process and watching trends over time, as they compare to national quality trends, is very valuable. The involvement of bedside staff is necessary to assure "hard-wiring" of change into daily operations.

Maintaining Staff Safety While Reducing the Use of Seclusion and Restraints

Judy Rabinowitz, BS, RNC
Clinical Supervisor, Adult Behavioral Health Services

Jody Kapustka, BS, RNC
Clinical Supervisor, Adolescent Behavioral Health Services

Christine Krause, MS
Director, Behavioral Health Services
krausec@gmc.com

Mary Greeley Medical Center—Ames, Iowa

Editors' pick:

INSIGHTS & IDEAS FROM THIS FACILITY

Recognized national benchmarks demonstrated room for improvement, even with a long-standing QI program.

Facility Summary

Facility	Mary Greeley Medical Center—Ames, Iowa **www.mgmc.org**
Facility setting	Mary Greeley Medical Center, a community-based hospital, provides general medical and surgical care, intensive coronary care, medical telemetry, oncology, maternal and child services, behavioral health and acute rehab, and skilled nursing services. Outpatient services include but are not limited to ambulatory care service, home health, hospice, dialysis in three communities as well as radiation oncology services in two communities.
Teaching status	Non-teaching hospital
Ownership status	Municipal hospital owned by the City of Ames, Iowa
Community demographics	• Population 52,319 (2004); an increase of 4.7% since the 2000 census. • Average median age is 23.6. • Median household income for Ames is $36,042 and the unemployment rate is 3.2% (2005). • Primary industries in the Ames area include: services (health, legal, repair, lodging)—28.6%; public administration (government)—21.7%; and retail trade (grocery, auto, clothes, restaurant)—14.5%.
Number of hospital staffed beds	198
Indicators used	Nursing Hours per Patient Day, Falls, Pressure Ulcers, Physical/Sexual Assaults
System or unit improved	Unit-based improvements: reduction of restraint and seclusion use while maintaining or reducing injury assault rates to staff
Indicator(s) improved	Adult psychiatric/injury assault rates
QI report card/ document used	See Table 1 which is adapted from NDNQI Report
NDNQI participant since	Mary Greeley began submitting in January 2003. Behavioral health unit began submitting in January 2005.
Magnet™ status (include if applying)	Currently in review and documenting phase and plan to submit July 2007.

UNIT PROFILE

Unit size and type	Behavioral health services includes: • 15-bed acute inpatient adult unit • Distinctly separate seven-bed acute inpatient adolescent unit • Adult and adolescent intensive outpatient programs • Transitional living program which is a six-bed, home-like environment for adults with mental illness that transitions them from acute inpatient care into the community
Unit RN staff profile	RNs only: Average experience in behavioral health services at facility = 12.64 years • Education: 68% AA degree, 14% diploma, 18% BSN, 0% Graduate/PhD, 14% other Bachelors degree, 18% other Masters degree • 45% full-time status, 32% regular part-time status (40–80 hours per two-week pay period), 23% part-time status (less than 40 hours per two-week pay period) • 32% ANCC certified in psychiatric and mental health nursing
Skill mix of RNs, other personnel	Although separate units, the adult and adolescent inpatient staff are combined in this following: • Day shift (0700–1500): 11.5 FTEs of which 17.4% are management (both of whom are RNs); 26% are RNs; 17.4 % are unlicensed assistive personnel; 8.7% are clerical staff; and 30.4% are licensed social work staff • Evening shift (1500–2300): 5 FTEs of which 60% are RNs and 40% are unlicensed assistive personnel • Night shift (2300–0700): 3.0 FTEs of which 67% are RNs and 23% are unlicensed assistive personnel
Organizational structure of unit	Behavioral health services consists of a shared decision-making structure in areas of customer service/quality improvement, standards, practice, and education in which staff nurses, unlicensed assistive personnel, and licensed social work staff directly report to RN clinical supervisors within each of the adult or youth services continuums. The supervisors report to the director of behavioral health services who reports to the vice president. The vice president reports to the chief executive officer.

Maintaining Staff Safety While Reducing the Use of Seclusion and Restraints

Judy Rabinowitz, BS, RNC
Clinical Supervisor, Adult Behavioral Health Services

Jody Kapustka, BS, RNC
Clinical Supervisor, Adolescent Behavioral Health Services

Christine Krause, MS
Director, Behavioral Health Services
krausec@gmc.com

Introductory Summary: Looking Back

In August of 1999, the Centers for Medicare and Medicaid Services (CMS) released its Conditions of Participation (COPs) that significantly restricted the use of restraint and seclusion methods on patients. Beginning January 1, 2001, the Joint Commission on Accreditation of Healthcare Organizations (JCAHO) began surveying hospital's with new restraint and seclusion standards directed at determining evidence of compliance with the CMS rule. Mary Greeley Medical Center (MGMC), like many providers, was faced with the need to redefine its standard of care. The proposed changes would challenge the Inpatient Behavioral Health Unit's practice at MGMC. This prompted a quality initiative to review and revise existing processes and implement the new requirements with an intended outcome of reducing the use of restraint and seclusion on patients.

Mary Greeley Medical Center is a 220-licensed-bed regional, referral hospital located in central Iowa. As part of the continuum of behavioral health care, the organization has a 15-bed locked adult unit and an 8-bed locked adolescent unit. The decision by the medical center's behavioral health leadership team was to fully embrace the intent of the new rule that patients have the right to be free of restraints. The team set out to revise the standard of care for use of restraint and seclusion in the inpatient setting with a goal of providing an environment that minimizes the use of restraint and seclusion, ensures patient and staff safety, and invests resources to support this practice.

The most challenging issue that faced the organization was the "one-hour rule," which required that any patient who was restrained or secluded must be evaluated by a licensed independent practitioner within one hour of initiation of the restraint or seclusion. This was a significant challenge for MGMC because it did not maintain psychiatrists in the facility at all times. Additionally, members of the behavioral health medical staff believed that the reduction in use of restraint and seclusion would contribute to increased numbers and severity of assaults by patients upon staff. Staff members also expressed concern in shifting from an environment that authorized discretion in the use of restraint and seclusion to one in which using such methods is permitted only as a last resort after numerous other interventions have been tried and with a goal to decrease its overall use.

Revised Standard of Care

The revision of the restraint and seclusion standard of care was addressed through an established organizational improvement process at MGMC. The FOCUS-PDCA format (Plan-Do-Check-Act) was used to initiate the effort in late 2000 and is a continuous improvement process still used in ongoing efforts to reduce or eliminate our use of restraint and seclusion.

Initially the focus was on implementing the new standards and knowing and understanding restraint and seclusion usage (i.e., incidences, hours per incidence, incidences per shift, staff initiating). Once a baseline of utilization was established, strategies were implemented to focus on overall reduction of usage. The following changes were implemented from 2001–2004:

- Established a process to provide face-to-face physician assessment using the 24/7 in-house hospitalist,

- Revised the restraint and seclusion guideline to reflect the new process and CMS and JCAHO standards,

- Developed and implemented a clinical pathway and flow sheet for the restraint and seclusion process which would serve a dual purpose as a checklist and documentation tool (Figure 2),

- Developed and implemented a patient and family education brochure to be reviewed upon admission,

- Modified the admission process to include identification of high-risk medical conditions, developmental and gender issues, ethnicity, and history of abuse which might affect how a person reacts to physical contact as well as any prior history of restraint or seclusion and strategies that may have worked for the patient in the past to maintain or regain control,

- Developed and implemented an incident debriefing form,

- Developed and implemented mandatory de-escalation and violent patient management training for all staff within six months of hire and a minimum of annual review thereafter, including additional ongoing training and competency assessment to be conducted in areas such as physical application of restraint, restraint and seclusion policy and procedure, and monitoring of patients in restraint and seclusion,

- Increased utilization of therapeutic interventions and activities and camera monitoring,

- Gained input from persons served in cooperation with the local chapter of the National Alliance for the Mentally Ill, and

- Established new quality improvement restraint and seclusion data collection systems.

Behavioral Health Restraint and Seclusion Data

The process improvements implemented since 2001 have been effective in reducing our overall utilization of restraint and seclusion on patients. Mary Greeley Medical Center's restraint and seclusion use with patients has declined over 50% (Figure 1). More remarkable is the near elimination of restraint use. Internal data collected and reviewed quarterly on the use of restraint and seclusion indicates that the facility has only restrained three adolescents in the last three years and three adults in the last year. In the last three years, the facility's use of seclusion with adolescents

Transforming Nursing Data Into Quality Care:
Profiles of Quality Improvement in U.S. Healthcare Facilities

continues to be reduced and seclusion with adults has stabilized but has not declined. With the overall decline in utilization of restraint and seclusion, quarterly data are now more focused on hours per incident rather than tracking numbers of patients who are restrained or secluded. Similar to all inpatient settings, this is in an environment with continued reductions in length of stay and increased patient acuity.

Quality Measurement and Reporting: Staff Assault Data and the Addition of NDNQI

Over the course of this quality initiative to reduce the use of restraint and seclusion on patients, staff assaults were monitored quarterly through an employee variance report system. One of the original concerns of the behavioral health medical staff was that as the use of restraint and seclusion was decreased, the injuries to staff by patient assault would increase. Employee injury records kept at the medical center indicate that assaults and assaults with injuries have not increased.

MGMC had been using the National Database of Nursing Quality Indicators (NDNQI) to benchmark performance on numerous indicators throughout the facility since January 2003. In 2004, it was brought to the attention of the behavioral health leadership team that there existed an NDNQI indicator related to assaults. The facility had collected and monitored the restraint and seclusion and staff assault data internally for a number of years and this would provide the opportunity for benchmarking with an external data source. While our performance had improved internally without the increase of assaults to staff, the more critical question was: How do we compare to other organizations of similar size and type? MGMC began submitting data to NDNQI for staff assaults in the first quarter of 2005 (Table 1). After several reporting periods, the behavioral health leadership began to note that while our assaults with injuries had improved in comparison to the unit's data, there appeared to be room for

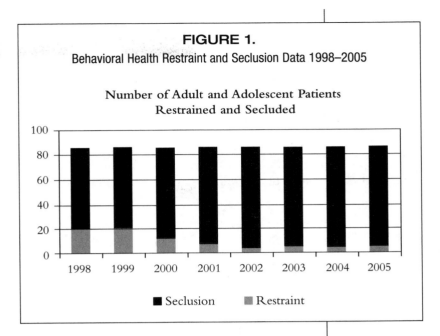

FIGURE 1.

Behavioral Health Restraint and Seclusion Data 1998–2005

Number of Adult and Adolescent Patients Restrained and Secluded

improvement as indicated by comparison to the "all facility data."

Quality Improvement: Continuous Improvement

Over the course of the ensuing quarters, the data indicated that the medical center continued to demonstrate improvement in injuries associated with assaults. The NDNQI data have challenged us to improve our performance related to the external benchmark, a goal we would not have envisioned had we just continued with the internal comparison. Through a continued FOCUS-PDCA approach, numerous strategies have been implemented over the course of the last year which have helped to improve the safety of the environment, including:

- Implementation of a self-soothing cart to provide activities and resources for patients to use to assist in modulating their own behavior,

- Closer monitoring by supervisors of staffing needs and increasing to 1:1 staffing with at-risk patients,

TABLE 1.

NDNQI Injury Assault Rates for Mary Greeley Medical Center for 2005 and Q1-06

	Q1-2005	Q2-2005	Q3-2005	Q4-2005	Q1-2006	Avg.
Adult and Adolescent Behavioral Health Unit	5.65	1.13	1.19	0.00	0.00	1.59

(Injury Assault Rates represent a subset of total assault rates per 1,000 patient days.)

National Comparative Information—Bedsize, All Facilities

10th Percentile	0.00	0.00	0.00	0.00	0.00	0.00
25th Percentile	0.00	0.00	0.00	0.00	0.00	0.00
50th Percentile	0.65	0.42	0.00	0.62	0.00	0.34
75th Percentile	1.88	1.60	1.19	1.42	1.28	1.47
90th Percentile	3.69	3.42	2.68	3.37	2.35	3.10
# of Reporting Units	75	118	144	170	171	136

(The lower the percentile ranking, the better the performance.)

- Education for staff on diagnostic-specific symptoms and improved treatment strategies (i.e., dissociative identity disorder, borderline personality disorder, trauma models of care), and

- Additional training for staff regarding unit safety and self-defense strategies.

Quality Improvement: Use of Standardized Databases

Databases that provide comparative data related to the inpatient behavioral health environment are limited, and the NDNQI database has provided MGMC behavioral health services a means of comparative analysis with similar institutions to track our outcomes related to employee assaults. In the future, the NDNQI measure will offer behavioral health providers much needed access to benchmark performance data to determine the success or failure of critical patient and staff safety outcomes which are under intense scrutiny in the current health care environment.

Lessons Learned

As with any quality improvement initiative, the improvement in outcomes is not seen in the first quarter and not likely even in the second, but is seen over time, perhaps one or two years later. In this particular process, the impact of our work was not really seen for almost three years. Diligence is important by continuing to keep the end goal in mind. Another lesson in quality improvement that we realized in this journey was that you cannot rely on your assumptions. What was clearly an assumption, that assaults would increase if restraint and seclusion decreased, was proven wrong. If we had continued to embrace this assumption we would not have made the changes that improved this outcome for our patients.

The intervention that provided the greatest positive impact in this process improvement was implementation of mandatory training for our staff in the area of managing aggressive behavior. Prior to requiring this education, it was not uncommon to observe staff employing strategies that escalated patient behavior. In our current environment, escalation is rare and when it is evident, staff employ strategies to actively de-escalate the behavior. This educational program has an approximate annual cost of $8,000 to train about 60 staff.

Conclusions and Implications

The NDNQI Database has provided Mary Greeley Medical Center a means of benchmarking facility performance. It has been used to demonstrate that the revisions implemented in the standard of care to minimize the use of restraint and seclusion have not further jeopardized staff safety, as was the initial concern. The

FIGURE 2.
Clinical Pathway and Flowsheet for Restraint and Seclusion Process

Pre-Restraint / Seclusion		Initial			Initiation of Restraint/Seclusion		Initial			Monitoring		Initial			Release / Debriefing		Initial		
Date:		11	7	3	Date:		11	7	3	Date:		11	7	3	Date:		11	7	3
Time:					Time:					Time:					Time:				

Pre-Restraint / Seclusion

Behavior observed:_____
_____
_____
_____
_____
_____
_____
_____
_____
_____
_____
_____

Least restrictive interventions attempted:
[ ] patient time out
[ ] relaxation techniques
[ ] 1:1 interv with staff
[ ] diversional activities
[ ] 1:1 nursing care
[ ] stress reduction activity
[ ] offer prescribed meds
[ ] verbal de-escalation
[ ] re-direct patient focus
[ ] other, describe_____
_____
_____
_____
_____

11 7 3

Initiation of Restraint/Seclusion

Documentation of clinical justification:
[ ] Threatened self harm
[ ] Threatened harm to others
[ ] Harmed self
[ ] Harmed others
Describe pt's actions:
_____
_____
_____

Rationale for type of restraint chosen:
_____
_____
_____

[ ] Initiate restraint
[ ] Initiate seclusion
[ ] Psychiatrist's order obtained within 1hr (see R/S order label).
[ ] Immediately call Dr._____ for face-to-face assessment (time_____).

11 7 3

Monitoring

[ ] **Monitor on initiation and every 15 min (see Monitor Flowsheet).**
[ ] Dr._____ face to face assess completed within 1hr by (time_____).
4th Hour: Time_____
Evaluation by RN_____
_____
_____

[ ] Called psychiatrist for writtn/verbal order (time_____).
[ ] Psychiatris order obtained (see restraint / seclude order).

7th Hour: Time_____
[ ] **Continue monitoring every 15 min (see Monitor Flowsheet).**
Re-evaluation by RN_____
_____
_____

[ ] Called Dr._____ for face-to-face assess (time_____).
[ ] Order received.
[ ] Call psychiatrist for face to face assess. (time_____)

End of 8th Hour:
[ ] Call psychiatrist for written/verbal renewal order (time_____).
[ ] Psychiatrist order obtained (see restraint/ seclude label).
[ ] Dr._____ completed face-to-face assess (time_____).

11 7 3

Release / Debriefing

Release time_____

Cumlative hours in restraints_____

[ ] Pt invited to debriefing
[ ] Family invited to debriefing (names:
_____
_____
)
[ ] Pt refused to attend.
[ ] Family refused to attend.
Debriefing:
Date_____
Time_____
[ ] Debriefing conducted within 24 hours of release from R/S. (See debriefing form.)
[ ] Recommended changes to tx plan:
_____
_____
_____

11 7 3

Initials	Signature/Title	Initials	Signature/Title

MARY GREELEY MEDICAL CENTER Ames, Iowa

CLINICAL PATH: TREATMENT PLAN MODIFICATION
RESTRAINT/SECLUSION-ADULT -- Behavioral Health

Physical/Sexual Assaults:
Maintaining Staff Safety While Reducing the Use of Seclusion and Restraints

database has also encouraged further improvements in nursing practice in our behavioral health setting.

Members of the behavioral health leadership team have recently attended continuing education in the area of "trauma informed care." Sessions have focused on creating an environment that promotes client empowerment and education in self-modulation of aggressive behaviors. Such strategies have over time led to the complete elimination of restraint use in facilities that have embraced and practiced these models. MGMC will soon initiate a complete physical remodeling of its inpatient behavioral health facilities with plans to incorporate some of these concepts. The plan includes the addition of a comfort room which will incorporate design elements and hands-on tools for clients to learn and practice these techniques. Our continuous improvement efforts will continue as we strive to be a restraint-free facility.

Patient Falls

Defined:

A patient fall is an unplanned descent to the floor (or extension of the floor, e.g., trash can or other equipment) with or without injury to the patient, and occurs on an eligible reporting nursing unit. All types of falls are to be included whether they result from physiological reasons (fainting) or environmental reasons (slippery floor). Include assisted falls — when a staff member attempts to minimize the impact of the fall.

Exclude falls by:

• Visitors

• Students

• Staff members

• Patients on units not eligible for reporting

• Patients from eligible reporting unit, however patient was not on unit at time of the fall (e.g., patient falls in radiology department)

Injury Falls:

The extent of injury is based upon the patient's condition 24 hours later.

Formula:

Total Falls: (Number of Patient Falls X 1000)/Total Number of Patient Days

Injury Falls: (Number of Patient Injury Falls X 1000)/Total Number of Patient Days

National Injury Fall Rate Benchmarks Motivate Cycles of Nursing Process Improvement

Tammi Erving-Mengel, RN, MSN, CNAA, BC
Vice President Inpatient Nursing
High Point Regional Health System
tmengel@hprhs.com

High Point Regional Health System—High Point, North Carolina

Editors' pick:

INSIGHTS & IDEAS FROM THIS FACILITY

Developed a method for communicating patient fall risks to all healthcare staff, which proved helpful.

Facility Summary

Facility	High Point Regional Health System—High Point, North Carolina **www.highpointregional.com**
Facility setting	The triad region of central North Carolina
Teaching status	Non-teaching
Ownership status	Private, nonprofit
Community demographics	The Health System serves a primary and secondary service area of approximately 422,583 people; 163,210 in the primary service area and 259,373 in the secondary service area. The three largest ethnic groups served are: Caucasian (60%), African American (32%), and Hispanic (5%).
Number of hospital staffed beds	384
Indicators used	Patients falls and patient falls with injury
System or unit improved	System-wide improvement across all units
QI report card/ document used	• NDNQI • Departmental scorecards
NDNQI participant since	December 2003
Magnet™ status	Magnet designation 2001; Magnet re-designation 2005

UNIT PROFILE

Unit size and type	Four units are profiled. • 7 North is a 30-bed medical unit • OCU is an 18-bed medical oncology unit • 6 North is a 36-bed med–surg unit (orthopedics, gastrointestinal, urology) • 5 South is a 30-bed med–surg unit (female patients only with a small pediatric population)
Unit RN staff profile	Associate degree nurses make up approximately 54% (429) of the RN staff on the med–surg units, while 44% (365) of the RN staff are BSN-prepared
Unit skill mix of RNs, other personnel	The skill mix is predominantly RNs and nursing assistants. The units profiled have 30 to 36 beds each and the nurse–patient ratio is generally 1:6. The nursing assistant role is a support role to the RN staff. Each nursing assistant is typically assigned to two nurses and cares for approximately eight patients on the day shifts.
Organizational structure of unit	The staff members of these units have a shift manager (unit coordinator) who is responsible for the activities of the shift. A performance coach has responsibility for the unit and staff performance around the clock. The performance coach reports to a director. The director has oversight responsibility for two to four units.

National Injury Fall Rate Benchmarks Motivate Cycles of Nursing Process Improvement

Tammi Erving-Mengel, RN, MSN, CNAA, BC
Vice President Inpatient Nursing
High Point Regional Health System
tmengel@hprhs.com

Introductory Summary

High Point Regional Hospital is a licensed 384-bed, private, nonprofit facility. Included in the bed complement are 24 behavioral health beds, and 30 subacute beds. The remainder of beds are allocated for acute services, with 102 assigned for critical care or intermediate critical care. The medical staff is composed of over 200 physicians. The hospital staff consists of 2,204 full-time and part-time employees, with 794 of those employees being Registered Nurses. Over 350 volunteers give generously of their time to support hospital activities and services.

High Point Regional Health System (HPRHS) serves a primary and secondary service area of approximately 422,583 people; 163,210 in the primary service area and 259,373 in the secondary service area. The three largest ethnic groups served by HPRHS are: Caucasian (60 %), black/African American (32 %) and Hispanic (5%). Primary service lines include cardiac, neuroscience, oncology, orthopedics, behavioral health, and women's health. Located in the Triad Region of North Carolina, the HPRHS community is bordered by two larger cities, each a 20-mile drive. These cities are served by four other nonprofit health systems including one major medical center with an affiliated medical school. The closest hospital is 10 miles away in a smaller city.

The HPRHS nursing staff received Magnet Designation in June 2001 and re-designation in 2005.

NDNQI Startup Considerations

High Point Regional Health System has participated in NDNQI since December 2003. It was believed that participation in NDNQI would provide HPRHS the opportunity to benchmark with other Magnet facilities and facilities striving for Magnet designation. Collection and reporting of data was done, however, without comparative data, there was no knowledge regarding best practice. Participation in NDNQI was important because it compared our results to other facilities that had been recognized for nursing excellence. It was important to the nursing leadership council and staff to benchmark with facilities that had been recognized as Magnets. We believed this would help us to achieve our vision to be the best place for patients to receive care.

Every nursing unit eligible to submit data is participating in the database. Pressure ulcer prevalence, patient falls, and nursing hours per patient day are the predominant indicators that data are submitted for. HPRHS recently served as a pilot test site for the new physical restraint prevalence indicator.

The units profiled in this paper are two medical surgical units and two medical units. The nursing staff provides care to a variety of surgical patients including orthopedic, urologic, vascular and gastrointestinal. They also care for patients with medical conditions such as acute and chronic lung disease, neurological disorders/disease, renal disease and cancer. The skill mix is predominantly Registered Nurses and Nursing Assistants. The units profiled have 30 to 36 beds each, and the nurse to patient ratio is generally 1:6. The nursing assistant role is a support role to the RN staff. Each nursing assistant is typically assigned to two nurses and cares for approximately eight patients on the day shifts.

Staff members and nursing leadership were excited about participation in this database. Benchmarking data related to nursing-sensitive indicators had not been available to the us at the individual department level. Data collection related to pressure ulcers, falls, and nursing hours per patient day had been collected and reported using internal benchmarks. We believed that we had good patient outcomes and we also believed that participation in a comparative data base would validate our beliefs.

When the decision was made to use the NDNQI database and this decision was shared with staff, it was believed that all nursing departments at HPRHS would have results in the most positive quartiles. As data were submitted and results were returned, this optimism turned to realism and the desire to improve began to emerge.

Quality Measurement and Reporting

Participation in the NDNQI database provided HPRHS benchmarking information related to the total number of patient falls and rates of patient falls with injury. Initially, this information was shared through the Nursing Performance Improvement Team (NPIT) and the Nursing Leadership Council. The NDNQI reports were distributed to these teams and then to the nursing units.

The nursing staff at HPRHS has always prided themselves on providing exceptional patient care and the data from NDNQI indicated some opportunities for improvement. The benchmarking data revealed that the rate of falls at HPRHS was either at the mean or higher than other hospitals in the database. This information created a sense of urgency to improve.

Information was shared with other members of the nursing staff. This created interest on the part of the other clinical teams (Research and Clinical Practice) to assist in making improvements. Members of the Research Team reviewed current literature to gain knowledge of what tools were available to screen patients for risk of falls and the cost (financial and human suffering) associated with patient falls that result in injury. The Research Team recommended that HPRHS adopt the Morse Falls scale to determine patient risk for falls. The Clinical Practice Team agreed with the recommendation and a subcommittee was created to develop the policy, documentation tool, and plan of care template and determine the method for education and implementation. Use of the Morse Falls scale was implemented in December 2004. The total number of falls did not seem to decrease (Figures 1, 2). Evaluation of this trend revealed that the fall risk assessments were being done; however there was poor communication about the level of fall risk between nurses and no communication of risk to other healthcare providers. It was felt that there was an opportunity to improve by creating a process that would promote identification of fall risk, communication of the risk, and implementation of protective measures.

In the winter of 2005, the organization began work on a quality framework that would align the goals of individual employees with their department and the organization goals. This was done by creating a balanced scorecard that is based on the strategic plan. Each department also developed a scorecard that identified outcomes for the department and what contributions the department makes to the organization. Each indicator on the scorecard had a target goal and a stretch goal identified. The target goal established should be accomplished within a year timeframe. Stretch goals are identified as three year goals. The nursing-sensitive indicators are placed on the scorecard for each nursing department, including the rates for total patient falls and patient falls with injury. The nursing-sensitive indicator goals were established using the information obtained from the NDNQI quarterly reports. The mean is often used as the target goal and the appropriate upper or lower quartile score is used for the stretch goal. These scorecards were implemented in October 2005. The outcome data on each scorecard provide staff information about the performance of their department.

Quality Improvement

During the spring and summer of 2005, two falls occurred that resulted in significant injury to the patient. The falls occurred on two different units, creating an organizational concern about how patient risk for falls was assessed and managed. These falls created the following questions:

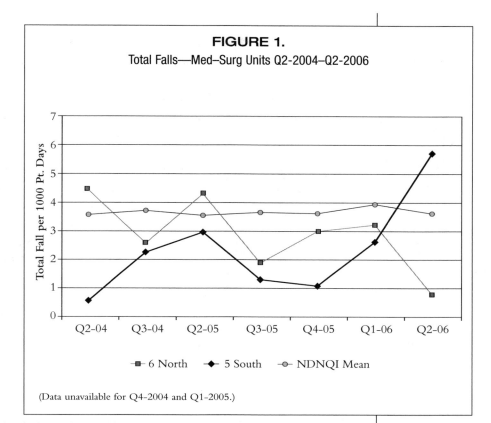

FIGURE 1.
Total Falls—Med–Surg Units Q2-2004–Q2-2006

(Data unavailable for Q4-2004 and Q1-2005.)

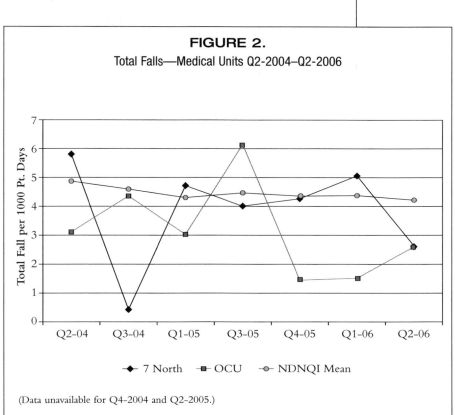

FIGURE 2.
Total Falls—Medical Units Q2-2004–Q2-2006

(Data unavailable for Q4-2004 and Q2-2005.)

FIGURE 3.
Fall Prevention and Management Program—The Stoplight

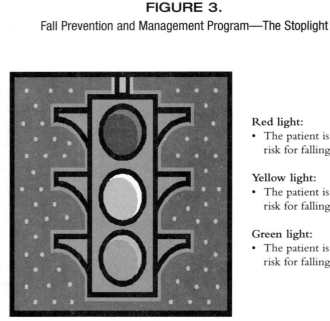

Red light:
- The patient is at high risk for falling

Yellow light:
- The patient is at low risk for falling

Green light:
- The patient is not at risk for falling

- Understanding the definition of fall and near fall,
- Employee responsibility in fall prevention,
- Assessment of risk for falls,
- Implementation of "stoplight" method (Figure 3) to identify the patient's risk level,
- Implementation of fall prevention strategies, and
- Staff response when a fall occurs.

There were two key components of the fall prevention and management plan. The use of a stoplight to identify the risk level of each patient and the performance of an environmental assessment after a fall has occurred. Stoplight signs were developed to be placed on the door of every patient room after the Morse Falls Screen was done. A red stoplight indicates a high risk, yellow indicates low risk, and green indicates no risk for falls. These signs are seen by everyone and education to the entire hospital staff included what to do when seeing a patient at high risk attempt to get out of bed (or a chair) without assistance. The team also developed "stoplight badges" to be placed on the patient's clothing when leaving the unit for a test or procedure. This communicates to the transporter and to the receiving department the level of risk for falls.

The environmental assessment that takes place if a fall occurs is done by a team consisting of the nursing supervisor, environmental services supervisor, and a staff member from the facilities department. They review the events leading up to the fall and then examine the area the fall occurred to determine if any environmental hazards could have been prevented. This information is being tracked and analyzed for trends. A future goal is to track "near falls" and identify any environmental issues that may be causing falls or near falls. The Fall Prevention and Management Team continues to meet and monitor the data. Changes to the plan will be proposed and implemented based on data trends. Each nursing department continues to monitor patient falls with injury on the departmental scorecards and the NDNQI comparative information is used to help establish benchmarks.

- What happens after the patient's risk for falls is determined?
- How do others know what the patient's risk for falls is?
- Who is responsible for fall prevention?

In the fall of 2005, working collaboratively with the Risk Management Department, an interdisciplinary team was formed to do a "failure mode and effect analysis" on falls. The data showed that there had been almost no change in the rate of patient falls over the course of three years. The goal of this team was to develop a process that would reduce the number of falls and eliminate falls that caused serious injury.

In March 2006, the team rolled out the "Fall Prevention and Management Plan." This plan requires that every employee be involved in preventing falls and keeping patients safe. The plan is based on six components:

Lessons Learned

Implementation of a comprehensive fall prevention program has been a lengthy process. We believed that use of a risk assessment scale to identify risk for falls would create awareness and promote preventive measures. We found that this was not necessarily true. While it raised awareness of the nursing staff after initial implementation, it was not sustained. It also did not communicate a patient's risk for falls to other care providers. We discovered that we needed to put a process in place that communicated the patient risk for falls. This process had to be visible to everyone who came in contact with patients.

The education of staff was done through a "cascade learning" process. We produced education packets (that included data related to falls) that described the process for identifying risk for falls and how to respond when confronted a high-risk patient attempting to move without assistance. The information was given to managers and supervisors who then shared the information with their staff. Each department was given four weeks to educate staff, at which time the use of the stoplights began. As this process was implemented, managers of the nursing units ensured that the stoplights were being placed on each patient door as the risk assessment was done. We continue to monitor each room to ensure that we are communicating risk for falls to all care providers. As we implemented the use of the stoplights, we also placed "patient safety signs" in each patient room. These signs explained to the patients and families what the stoplights were for and how to ensure safety. An interesting use of the

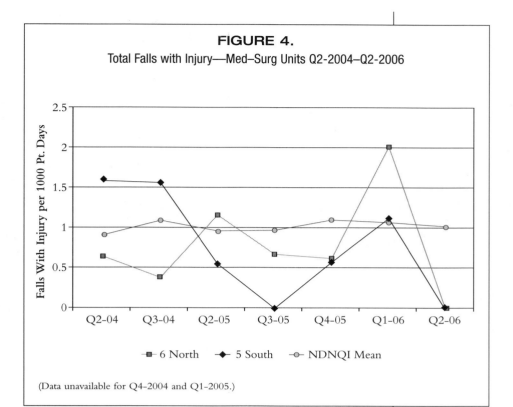

FIGURE 4.

Total Falls with Injury—Med–Surg Units Q2-2004–Q2-2006

(Data unavailable for Q4-2004 and Q1-2005.)

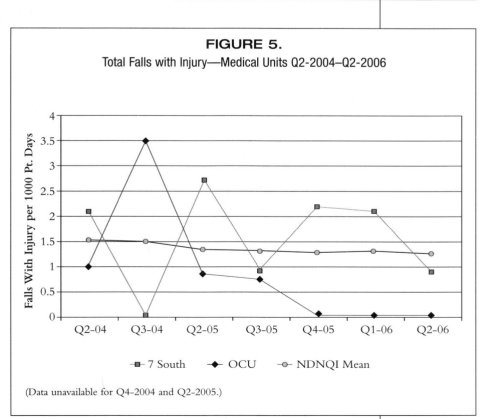

FIGURE 5.

Total Falls with Injury—Medical Units Q2-2004–Q2-2006

(Data unavailable for Q4-2004 and Q2-2005.)

stoplights occurred on the postpartum unit. A visitor was seen changing a green stoplight to a red and then back to green a few hours later. When questioned why this was being done, he reported that the red stoplight was to indicate that the patient was resting and did not want visitors!

The cost of implementing this process was approximately $5,000 for the stoplights and for the stoplight badges. This does not include the salary costs for education. We will continue to analyze our falls, falls with injury, and the information obtained from the falls assessment team to determine any future changes to the process and to evaluate any actual or potential cost savings.

Results of the Fall Prevention and Management Plan are not clear at this point. The goal to reduce the number of falls with injury shows varied results, with some units decreasing their rates and others needing to stabilize their process (Figures 4, 5). We will continue to monitor and analyze our results and make changes to the plan as determined by the team.

Conclusions and Implications

The nursing staff at High Point Regional Health System will continue to participate in the NDNQI database to measure our results to other Magnet facilities. Having the NDNQI benchmark information encourages us to continue looking for methods to improve our care and ultimately our outcomes. Excellence at High Point Regional Health System is defined as being in the top decile. The goal of the nursing staff at HPRHS is to be the benchmark in all indicators of the NDNQI database.

NDNQI Data Provide Goals for Fall Prevention Action Plans

Patti Vanhook, APRN, MSN, BC
Magnet Coordinator
VanhookPM@MSHA.com

Myra Jones, RN, BSN
Clinical Policy & Procedure Coordinator

Johnson City Medical Center (JCMC)—Johnson City, Tennessee

Editors' pick:

INSIGHTS & IDEAS FROM THIS FACILITY

Persisted in order to fine-tune process improvements and get staff compliance and detailed elements of fall prevention.

Facility Summary

Facility	Johnson City Medical Center (JCMC)—Johnson City, Tennessee **www.MSHA.com**
Facility setting	• Level I Trauma Center—one of only six in Tennessee • Leading heart hospital in East Tennessee—recognized in 2004 and 2005 as one of the top 100 U.S. hospitals in cardiovascular services • Regional Cancer Center, which has clinical collaborations with Harvard, Duke, and Vanderbilt medical centers and St. Jude's Children's Research Hospital • Organ transplant program—only program in region • Perinatal Center—only state-designated unit in region • Hospital-based air ambulance service—only one in region • Magnet designation—first hospital in Tennessee to be authorized • Children's Hospital at JCMC, a member of NACHRI since 1992; North Side Hospital; Johnson City Specialty Hospital; James H. & Cecile C. Quillen Rehabilitation Hospital; and Woodridge Hospital behavioral care
Teaching status	Teaching hospital affiliated with Quillen College of Medicine at East Tennessee State University (ETSU)
Ownership status	Nonprofit
Community demographics	Predominantly Caucasian (94%) but multi-ethnic with 2.3% Black, 1.7% Hispanic, and less than 1% Native American and Pacific Islander population
Number of hospital staffed beds	503
Indicators used	Patient falls
System or unit improved	Unit improvement—patient falls
Indicator(s) improved	Falls per 1,000 pt. days
QI report card/ document used	Blueprint: Establishes and communicates goals and expectations of performance at all levels of the organization. The blueprint includes outcome measures for each pillar of the Performance Improvement House of Quality model: clinical effectiveness, operational effectiveness, stakeholder safety, and service excellence. Patient falls are reported under the stakeholder safety category.

NDNQI participant since	2002
Magnet™ status	Magnet facility

UNIT PROFILE

Unit size and type	• 20-bed medical–surgical • 17-bed renal unit for medical–surgical patients
Unit RN staff profile	• Age range: 24 to 54 years • Average experience: 15 years • Certified in specialty (med–surg): 2
Unit skill mix of RNs, other personnel	• Unit-7P: 3 RN, 1.5 UAP • Unit 7A: 2 RN, 2 LPN, 3 UAP • Clinical Nurse Specialist
Organizational structure of unit	Director of Strategic Service Unit Pulmonary, Renal, Oncology • Unit Manager • Clinical Leader • Shift Leader Director of Strategic Service Unit • Pulmonary, Renal, Oncology Unit Manager • Clinical Leader • Shift Leader

NDNQI Data Provide Goals for Fall Prevention Action Plans

Patti Vanhook, APRN, MSN, BC
Magnet Coordinator
VanhookPM@MSHA.com

Myra Jones, RN, BSN
Clinical Policy & Procedure Coordinator

Introductory Summary

Johnson City Medical Center (JCMC) is locally owned and is part of the 11-hospital system comprising the Mountain States Health Alliance (MSHA). JCMC is located in Johnson City, Tennessee, and has a service area that includes northeastern Tennessee, southwestern Virginia, southeastern Kentucky, and northwestern North Carolina. Since 1911, JCMC has been dedicated to serving people of this Appalachian region and assisting them to attain their highest possible level of health. JCMC, the second hospital built in Tennessee, has grown to a 503-bed, nonprofit, comprehensive, acute care teaching hospital affiliated with East Tennessee State University (ETSU) and ETSU's James H. Quillen College of Medicine.

The multi-ethnic population served by the medical center is considered mixed rural and urban. The area is predominantly Caucasian and has an increasing Hispanic population. In the past fiscal year, JCMC has provided care to 218,028 outpatients and 26,002 inpatients.

JCMC is also a medical major referral center providing Level I trauma care and hosts the region's only dedicated emergency medical air transport service. JCMC has the region's only full-service children's hospital, is a member of National Association of Children's Hospitals and Related Institutions (NACHRI) since 1992, has a Level 3 neonatal intensive care unit, and is affiliated with St. Jude's Children's Research Hospital, one of only four in the nation. A full range of specialty and subspecialty services, including organ transplantation and some of the most advanced diagnostic and surgical techniques, is available at the facility. Cardiovascular surgery is a major subspecialty, with JCMC being recognized as a Solucient Top 100 hospital in 2005. Our most prestigious recognition was being designated as the first Magnet hospital in Tennessee in January 2005.

FIGURE 1.

House of Quality

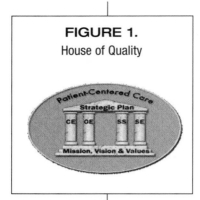

NDNQI Startup Considerations

As part of a multi-hospital system, Johnson City Medical Center subscribes to the system-wide approach to performance improvement. The Performance Improvement (PI) plan of Mountain States Health Alliance uses a leadership-driven, system-wide approach to achieving and sustaining excellence through continual performance measurement and performance improvement activities. These activities are collaborative and interdisciplinary, utilizing a philosophy which through teamwork allows MSHA to best improve its clinical outcomes, stakeholder safety, operational efficiency, and service excellence. An overarching environment of patient-centered care points to the need for ongoing performance improvement activity.

The framework of performance improvement activities and the methodology by which the PI plan is executed is the House of Quality concept (Figure 1).

The foundation of the PI plan comprises MSHA's mission, vision, and values. "Pillars" represent the four key elements around which all PI initiatives are prioritized. At the base of each pillar are the minimal performance standards for quality monitoring activities.

Pillars	Performance Standards (Minimum for Each)
Clinical Effectiveness (CE)	Maximizing patient outcomes
Operational Effectiveness (OE)	Creating value for our customers
Stakeholder Safety (SS)	"Do no harm," either through acts of omission or acts of commission
Service Excellence (SE)	Being the provider and employer of choice for ALL our customers, providing service through well-designed processes within a culture of care and respect

The "roof" of the House of Quality represents the MSHA strategic plan. The strategic goals and measures for MSHA are defined in this plan and provide the rationale for prioritizing and selecting performance improvement initiatives in each of the four pillars.

The PI process is completed using three distinct components performed in a continuous cycle (Figure 2).

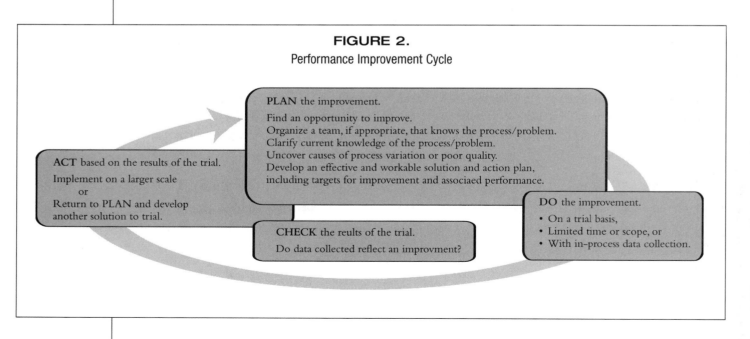

FIGURE 2.

Performance Improvement Cycle

PLAN the improvement.

Find an opportunity to improve.
Organize a team, if appropriate, that knows the process/problem.
Clarify current knowledge of the process/problem.
Uncover causes of process variation or poor quality.
Develop an effective and workable solution and action plan, including targets for improvement and associaed performance.

ACT based on the results of the trial.

Implement on a larger scale
or
Return to PLAN and develop another solution to trial.

CHECK the reults of the trial.

Do data collected reflect an improvment?

DO the improvement.

• On a trial basis,
• Limited time or scope, or
• With in-process data collection.

The Mountain States Health Alliance has a long history of using data to guide decision-making. The Chief Nursing Officer (CNO) realized that participation in NDNQI would give JCMC the opportunity to benchmark nationally for direct patient outcomes of nursing care. The CNO shared information about NDNQI with her nursing leaders and the Patient Care Practice Council and the Performance Improvement Training Council. The indicators JCMC selected for acute care include patient falls, pressure ulcer prevalence, skill mix, nursing hours per patient day, and the RN Job Satisfaction Survey. The indicators were selected based on the relevance of the indicators to the majority of the patient care areas at JCMC. The medical center joined the NDNQI database in 2002.

The prospect of benchmarking against similar units excited the leaders and the council membership. The council members focused their energy on the frontline nurses to educate them about nurse-sensitive indicators and measure patient outcomes related to nursing care. The nurses began to understand the value of data contributing to their patient care.

The JCMC fall prevention and intervention program was developed based on the following historical findings and premises:

- Patient fall risk increases exponentially after admission to the hospital. The average cost of a patient fall is $19,440 and 20–30% of the patients who fall suffer severe injuries, resulting in a decreased ability to ambulate, lower independence, and increased premature death (Hendrich 2005).

- Factors contributing to increased fall risk include medications that may create confusion, drop in blood pressure, gait instability (Cumming 1998; Moore and O'Keeffee, 1999), male gender, symptomatic depression, altered elimination, dizziness/vertigo, and inability to raise from a sitting to a standing position without assistance (Hendrich, Bender, Nyhuis 2003).

- There is a relationship between nurse hours per patient day (NHPPD) and patient falls (Dunton, Gajewski, Taunton, Moore 2004). These NDNQI data in this study were used to assess the relationship between NHPPD and patient falls. Their findings supported that increasing NHPPD up to 15 demonstrated a decrease in patient falls for medical, surgical, med–surg, and step-down units. An interesting finding in this study is that patient falls increased in relationship to the percentage of contract hours for medical–surgical units but not for all other nursing unit types ($p<.01$).

- Research demonstrates that only 78% of physiologic falls can be anticipated and prevented (Morse 1997).

- A process to assess patient risk on a continuum and assign fall prevention interventions has been demonstrated to decrease patient injury falls (Hendrich et al. 2003).

Quality Measurement and Reporting

In 2002, JCMC joined the NDNQI database enrolling the acute care units. Coinciding with this, the transitional care unit at JCMC began collaborating with other skilled units within Mountain States Health Alliance to decrease patient falls. They began by investigating the literature for best practices and identifying a comprehensive tool to assess fall risk. This project was multidisciplinary in nature, utilizing the expertise of frontline caregivers and a physical therapist. The program used the Hendrich Fall Model to assess risk on admission, designating a level of risk (low, medium, high); used a "traffic light" symbol to communicate risk (green = low, yellow = medium, and red = high); established interventions for each level of risk, including debriefing after each patient fall, and posting of a laminated "hand" symbol on the patient's door for those patients identified at risk. A trial program was implemented in February 2003. The success of the program was demonstrated by the decline in patient falls (Figure 3). These data were shared with the JCMC Patient Care

Practice Council and PI Training Council and the fall prevention program began known as Helping Hands. Admission history and assessment forms were changed throughout MSHA to include the Hendrich Fall Risk Assessment Model.

Quality Improvement: Planning, Data Collection, Discussion

The Patient Care Practice Council and the PI Training Council shared data from the transitional care units. They studied the data (Figure 4) and, based on increasing fall rates, the Unit 5500 PI team identified an opportunity for improvement.

The team began collecting data based on the Helping Hands fall prevention program. In this program, nurses post a laminated hand symbol on the door of patients at risk for falls. Most often patients were identified at risk after a fall. With the implementation of the Hendrich Fall Risk Model, the nurses had an objective means to identify patients at risk and post the helping hand proactively on admission. Data collection began with a small sample size of eight patients in February 2003.

2003 Trial: Data Indicators Used

- Fall risk data section appropriately completed upon admission

- Fall risk documented on plan of care

- Fall risk sign visible at patient's alcove

- Education on Helping Hands Program documented on patient's education record

- Helping Hands Program initiated if patient fell during admission

• • •

Fall risk data assessed on admission included: patient greater than 70 years of age; neurological disorders; his-

tory of previous falls; paralysis/weakness; dizziness/balance problems; confused/disoriented; taking sedatives/psychotropic/narcotics/diuretics; sensory impairment; and incontinence stool or urine. When two or more of these were checked, the Helping Hands program was implemented.

Data collection on these indicators provided a baseline to know where we were and identify ways to improve. Sample size was gradually increased (n=20 patients) through Q3-03. Poor compliance was reflected from the data collection on the indicators that were noted above.

Fall rates and results of data collection were discussed in staff meetings. In May and June 2003, team members participated in training sessions on how to prevent falls. Discussions that ensued during training identified a need for increased staff awareness regarding patient falls. During these discussions, it was learned that nurses considered restraining the patient a means of fall prevention. Also recognized was the need for increased compliance with all selected indicators. The staff were educated on the appropriate use of restraints according to the restraint protocol. The staff was required to ensure that restraints were being used appropriately according to the restraint protocol and not only as a means for fall prevention. Team members were anxious to decrease fall rates, provide quality patient care, and prevent injury and the potential for injury.

The fall risk assessment procedures were revised in September 2003 to include: recent history of falls (not slip/trip); altered elimination (incontinence, nocturia, frequency, urgency); confusion/disorientation; depression (symptomatic); dizziness/vertigo; poor mobility/generalized weakness; poor judgment (if not confused); and the choice of "other," allowing nurses to identify any other reason that a fall prevention program should be implemented. If any of the items were checked, the fall prevention program was implemented. The indicators utilized for data collection, as noted above, did not change with the revision in assessment for fall risk.

In October 2003, the clinical leader for Unit 5500, the risk manager for JCMC, and the Performance Improvement Training Council representative for Unit 5500 met to develop an action plan that would utilize the information obtained from the transitional nursing units project. The literature search for best practices was also reviewed. The resulting action plan to promote safety and decrease falls included the following steps:

- Patients were assessed for fall risk on admission and throughout their hospital stay.

- When fall risk was identified, "Fall Precaution" was to be noted on the clinical pathway in red ink.

- The Helping Hands symbol was to be placed in a visible location in the identified patient's alcove.

- The patient/family/significant other would be educated on the Helping Hands program by utilizing the program brochure. Completion of this step was to be documented on the interdisciplinary education record.

- "Bowel and bladder assistance every two hours" was to be noted on the clinical pathway in red ink.

- Documentation of "bowel and bladder assistance every two hours" was to be documented on the activity flow sheet.

Team members were sent again to training sessions to be re-educated on the revised action plan. Training

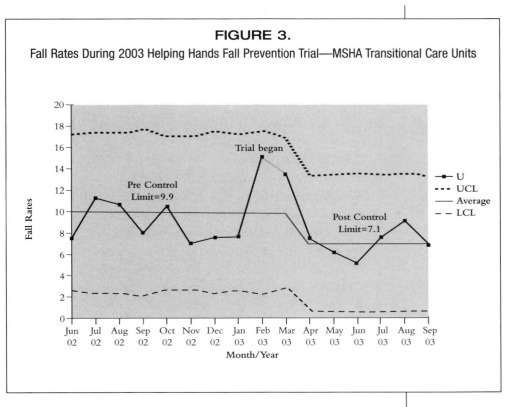

FIGURE 3.

Fall Rates During 2003 Helping Hands Fall Prevention Trial—MSHA Transitional Care Units

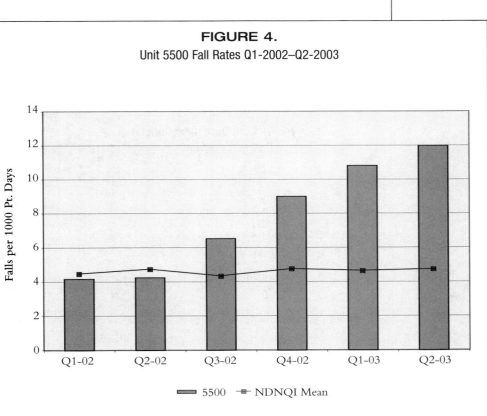

FIGURE 4.

Unit 5500 Fall Rates Q1-2002–Q2-2003

included a test to be completed by each team member. The test, which was a revision of a test developed for another unit at JCMC, covered information on the fall prevention program and proper use of restraints. The action plan was implemented in November 2003. Fall rates declined in Q4-03 (8.28/1,000 pt. days) to the rate in Q4-02 (9/1,000 pt. days).

Team members learned that a factor frequently contributing to patients' falls was their need for toileting assistance (e.g., increased need for toiletry). Therefore, an effort to establish critical thinking skills was begun with regards to the administration of certain medications; e.g. diuretics, laxatives, etc. During this time, team members requested more information on how to prevent patient falls and proactively identified those patients at high risk for falls.

Quality Improvement: Testing in Limited Trials

After assessing results of the 2003 trial program in the transitional care area, the PI team revised its data collection indicators. Beginning January 2004, data collection indicators reflected the action plan as follows:

January 2004 Trial: Data Indicators Used (First Revision)

- Fall risk assessment section completed on patient's initial history and assessment

- When fall risk identified, "Fall Precaution" noted on the clinical pathway in red ink

- Helping Hands symbol visibly located in patient's alcove

- Education on the Helping Hands brochure documented on interdisciplinary patient education record

- "Bowel and bladder assistance every two hours" noted on clinical pathway in red ink

- "Bowel and bladder assistance every two hours" documented on activity flow sheet

• • •

The sample size (n=120 patients) greatly increased with the data collection for first quarter 2004.

A new patient education information sheet—"Preventing Falls in the Hospital"—was developed by team members. The sheet was provided to patients who were alert, oriented, and could benefit from the information after being identified as a fall risk. Printed on brightly colored paper, the sheet was also available with other patient education materials in the hallway on Unit 5500. This allowed for easy access for visitors, patients, and team members. The clerical associate on Unit 5500 placed a copy of the patient education sheet on fall prevention within each admission packet for easy access for nursing staff on the unit. This practice was continued even after a newer brochure on fall prevention became available for MSHA in April 2005.

Even though fall rates declined by 38% (Figure 5) in the first quarter 2004, as compared to first quarter 2003, staff meetings continued to include discussions of fall rates and action plan progress. Journal articles on falls and patient safety were distributed to team members in April and May 2004. In June 2004, due to poor compliance with the new action plan, as evidenced by the data collected, team members were retrained on the new requirements. Team members were also required to complete a test on the action plan. The test increased awareness of criteria to use when assessing a patient's increased risk of falling, as well as providing specific examples of actions that could be implemented to prevent falls.

Fall rates declined 26.5% in second quarter 2004 as compared to those in second quarter 2003. In third quarter 2004, a poster on patient toileting rounds was placed in the Unit 5500 Team Conference Center (TCC) or nurses' station. Flyers printed on brightly colored paper were placed in each patient's alcove to remind team members to perform patient toileting rounds. Cards entitled "Pocket Reference for Fall Prevention" were also provided to team members. The cards included information related to the Hendrich Fall Risk Scale with a listing of possible interventions.

In third quarter 2004, nephrologists at JCMC requested that all renal failure patients not needing intensive care, progressive care, or transitional nursing facility care be housed on Unit 5500. The goal was to provide continuity of care for the dialysis patients. A shift leader for Unit 5500 was designated to serve as a liaison with bed placement nurses. New beds with low position and patient position alarm features were acquired. In-service education was provided to team members on the new beds.

In October and November 2004, data collection indicators were revised to reflect the change from the Helping Hands symbol to a colored traffic light symbol (green, yellow, or red). Through color coding, the new symbol more clearly denotes fall risk level. Therefore, red ink could no longer be used to document fall risk in the medical record. Data collection indicators were revised to reflect the action plan as follows:

November 2004 Trial: Data Indicators Used
(Second Revision)

- Fall risk assessment section completed on patient's initial H&P

- Appropriate fall risk symbol visibly located in patient's alcove

- Education on the Fall Prevention Program documented on interdisciplinary education record

- "Bowel and bladder assistance every two hours" documented on activity flow sheet

- Hendrich Fall Risk assessed every 24 hours on assessment flow sheet

• • •

Team members completed a computer-based learning module (CBL) on the Hendrich Fall Risk Scale, resulting in a request for clips to hang the paper traffic light symbols in patient alcoves.

In fourth quarter 2004, fall rates continued to decline, causing the PI team, once again, to revise the data collection indicators. Indicators were revised in January 2005 to reflect the change to the Hendrich Fall Risk Scale as follows:

January 2005 Trial: Data Indicators Used
(Third Revision)

- Fall risk assessed upon admission (Hendrich scale)

- Fall intervention flow sheet placed in patient's chart

- Fall intervention flow sheet documented appropriately

- Fall risk assessed daily (Hendrich scale)

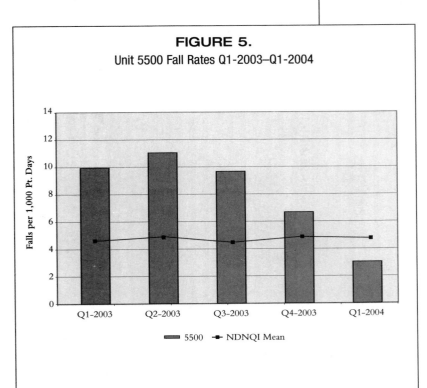

FIGURE 5.
Unit 5500 Fall Rates Q1-2003–Q1-2004

- Appropriate traffic light color posted visibly in patient's alcove

- Education on fall prevention documented on inter-disciplinary patient education record

• • •

Data collection in 2005 showed a gradual increase in compliance with some indicators. The PI team determined that it had been the frequent changes in policy and fall scales that had adversely affected the results of the data collection. Three different scales were used from 2003–2005 and team members expressed feeling overwhelmed by the constant changes in scales and policies. As soon as the team members become accustomed to one scale, the scale changed. However, team members were receptive to the need for the changes and wanted to maintain low fall rates and continually improve care. The NDNQI comparison data provided evidence of their efforts.

Team members anxiously awaited permanent traffic light signs for patient alcoves because the paper traffic lights were continually falling to the floor and being thrown away. In an effort to communicate with other disciplines, they attempted clipping the paper traffic lights on patients' charts, but the chart did not provide good visibility due to its location in the alcove. Efforts continued to improve the critical thinking skills with fall assessment and prevention (Figure 6).

In April 2005, Train the Trainer sessions were conducted on fall assessment, prevention, and intervention. The sessions educated team members who would then train other team members in their respective areas. Again, one of the data collection indicators had to be changed to reflect the placement of a laminated Fall Prevention Protocol in front of patients' charts, leading to team member frustration when the laminated protocols disappeared from patient charts. A paper copy of the protocol was placed on the charts by the clerical associate when a chart did not have the laminated protocol. Additional copies of the laminated protocol were also obtained and placed on charts when found to be missing.

To reinforce compliance with the PI team's recommendations, subsequent to the 2005 trial, Unit 5500 managers worked with staff members to set departmental and individual goals for fiscal year 2006. Departmental goals for fiscal year 2006 on Unit 5500 included meeting the comparative national mean for fall rate per 1,000 patient days. Individual goals for all Unit 5500 team members included completing patients fall assessment on admission and periodically thereafter.

In September 2005, a BSN management student from East Tennessee State University collected data on use of the patient movement alarms on the specialty beds as it relates to fall risk patients.

Data the student collected revealed team members were not setting the alarm for patients who were assessed as moderate to

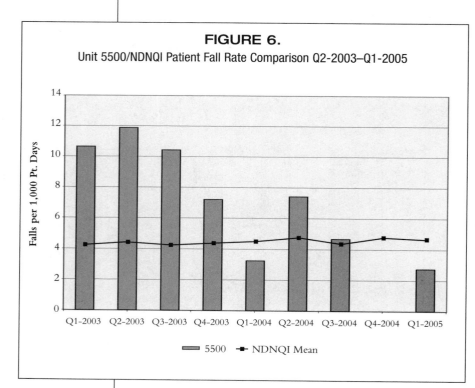

FIGURE 6.

Unit 5500/NDNQI Patient Fall Rate Comparison Q2-2003–Q1-2005

high risk for falls. The student provided training to team members on how bed alarms could reduce fall risk and how to set the bed alarms. A copy of instructions on how to set the bed alarms was posted in the Unit 5500 nurses station. Team members noted that after setting the bed alarms the alarm was not audible unless standing directly outside the patient's room with the door open. Biomedical engineering was called in to assist with troubleshooting and discovered a change in the patient call light system had affected the bed alarms. They began work to rectify the issue.

During fourth quarter 2005, additional training was provided to team members on preventing falls. This training introduced the team members to the Hendrich II Fall Scale, which was to be implemented in early 2006. Team members would also begin assessing fall risk every shift rather than only daily. A CBL module was also completed by all team members on the Hendrich II Fall Scale by February 2006.

Quality Improvement: Checking Trial Results

Fall rates declined through fourth quarter 2005 (Figure 7) even though data collection indicators did not show continual compliance with documentation. Improvement was noted, however, and the PI team agreed that the constant change had influenced team members' understanding of assessing patients for fall risk and documentation related to the indicators.

Quality Improvement: Acting to Produce a Final Action Plan

Permanent traffic light symbols (Figure 8) were posted in patient alcoves in January 2006. In March 2006, data collection indicators were modified to include fall risk assessment of patients for every shift.

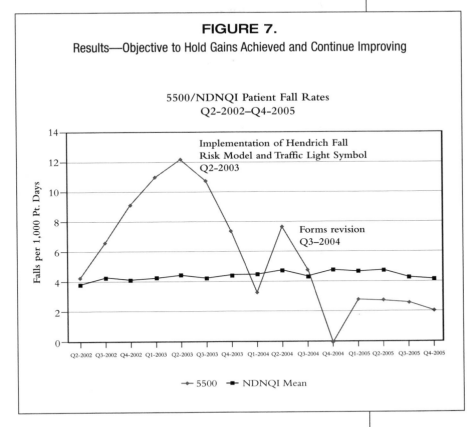

FIGURE 7.

Results—Objective to Hold Gains Achieved and Continue Improving

5500/NDNQI Patient Fall Rates
Q2-2002–Q4-2005

Implementation of Hendrich Fall Risk Model and Traffic Light Symbol Q2-2003

Forms revision Q3–2004

◆ 5500   ■ NDNQI Mean

Lessons Learned

Many lessons were learned throughout this process and the learning continues. Key lessons are noted below:

- Continual change in processes was frustrating for staff.

- Frontline nurses must observe that a procedure change is working in order to appreciate the value; i.e., data that demonstrated measurable outcome came six months after the practice change.

- Use of restraints does not decrease falls.

- Fall prevention is not just a nursing issue but involves all clinical and non-clinical care providers.

- A focused effort on reducing falls increased staff awareness of fall risk identification and implementation of efforts to decrease falls.

FIGURE 8.

Fall Prevention Traffic Light

- Individualizing the patient's plan of care to address fall risk is an important aspect of the program.

- Success with frontline empowerment is exciting and challenging.

Conclusions and Implications

Fall prevention is an interdisciplinary effort. One critical factor in fall prevention is the communication of the patient at risk. The installation and utilization of the traffic light signs and hard-wiring patient risk assessment have proven to be beneficial for this unit and for JCMC. Over time, Unit 5500 decreased patient fall rates from a high of 11.97/1,000 pt. days (second quarter 2003) to an average of 2.55/1,000 pt. days for calendar year 2005. JCMC ended the 2006 fiscal year with an overall patient fall rate of 2.88/1,000 pt. days. From the efforts on Unit 5500, a total of 12 patient falls can be estimated as having been prevented between the beginning of their initiative in second quarter 2003 to the final quarter of 2005. The savings in patient harm from injury is tremendous as is the financial savings for the hospital. According to Hendrich (2005) the average cost for a patient fall is $19,440 or a total potential savings of $233,280 for Unit 5500.

The efforts of this team were driven by the desire for change. In addition, the data from NDNQI provided the team with a realistic goal from comparable units caring for similar patients. The data from NDNQI continue to be used by this unit to benchmark their progress. During the first and second quarters of 2006, an increase in falls began to be noted. The clinical leader for the unit attributed an increase in the utilization of contract labor new to the facility and to her unit. The decrease in regular staffing and increase in temporary staffing are supported by the findings of Dunton, Gajewski, Taunton, and Moore (2004).

The fall program has been implemented throughout the Mountain States Health Alliance. The NDNQI data are reviewed on a quarterly basis by the Shared Leadership Council. This council is charged with the task of analysis of the data and working with individual units to form action plans as indicated.

References

American Nurses Association. *Scope and standards for nurse administrators (2nd Ed.)*. Washington, DC: Nursesbooks.org; 2004.

Ann Hendrich, Inc. Overview. Clayton, MO: http://www.ahendrichinc.com/falls/index.php; 2005. (Retrieved February 1, 2006)

Cumming RG. Epidemiology of medication-related falls and fractures in the elderly. *Drugs & Aging 1998;* 12(1):43-53.

Dunton N, et al. Nurse staffing and patient falls on acute care hospital units. *Nursing Outlook* 2004;52: 53-59.

Hendrich A, et al. Validation of the Hendrich II Fall Risk Model: a large concurrent case/control study of hospitalized patients. *Appl Nurs Res* 2003;16(1):9-21.

Moore AR, et al. Drug-induced cognitive impairment in the elderly. *Drugs & Aging* 1999;15(1):15-28.

Morse JM. *Preventing patient falls*. Thousand Oaks, CA: Sage Publications; 1997.

National Database of Nursing Quality Indicators. Washington, DC: American Nurses Association; 1998.

NDNQI Falls Data Support Decision Making by Nursing Leadership Councils on Equipment and Staff Education

Heidi Ritchie, RN, MS
Magnet Coordinator
heidi.ritchie@uhsinc.com

Carrie Shreck, RN, MS, CNAA-BC
Chief Nursing Officer

St. Mary's Regional Medical Center—Enid, Oklahoma

Editors' pick:

INSIGHTS & IDEAS FROM THIS FACILITY

*Sustained management effort
in order for successful adoption
of changes in nursing practices*

Facility Summary

Facility	St. Mary's Regional Medical Center—Enid, Oklahoma **www.stmarysregional.com**
Facility setting	Full complement of services with areas of specialization in cardiac services, neurosciences and neurosurgery, women's health, rehabilitation, emergency services, and outpatient services.
Teaching status	Non-teaching regional hospital
Ownership status	Universal Health Service, Inc.
Community demographics	Rural community of 48,000+ with a 2% growth rate. Home of Vance Air Force Base, Advance Food Company, oil, and farming industries. Campuses include: Northern Oklahoma College, Northwestern Oklahoma State University, and Autry Technology Center.
Number of hospital staffed beds	112
Indicators used	Nursing care hours, patient days, RN education, patient falls, pressure ulcers
System or unit improved	Unit improvements in each unit
Indicator(s) improved	Patient falls
QI report card/ document used	Nursing dashboard
NDNQI participant since	2002
Magnet™ status	Application submitted June 2006.

UNIT PROFILE

Unit size and type	• Med–Surg (Neuro): 20-bed unit • Rehabilitation: two units with 28 beds
Unit RN staff profile	• Med–Surg (Neuro): Mean RN age = 39; 76% of RNs full-time, 17% part-time, 6% per diem; 36% of RNs > 2 years on unit; 11% diploma, 45% ADN, 42% BSN • Rehabilitation: Mean RN age = 45; 71% full-time, 23% part-time, 5% per diem; 46% > 2 years on unit; 16% diploma, 41% ADN, 39% BSN
Unit skill mix of RNs, other personnel	• Med–Surg (Neuro): 50% of care hours provided by RNs, 20% by LPNs, 30% by NA/NT • Rehabilitation: 50% of care hours provided by RNs, 20% by LPNs, 30% by NA/NT
Organizational structure of unit	Each unit has predominantly RN staff in addition to LPNs and NA and US. Each unit has a RN clinical manager and both units report to the same RN director.

NDNQI Falls Data Support Decision Making by Nursing Leadership Councils on Equipment and Staff Education

Heidi Ritchie, RN, MS
Magnet Coordinator
heidi.ritchie@uhsinc.com

Carrie Shreck, RN, MS, CNAA-BC
Chief Nursing Officer

Introductory Summary

In 2001, the Risk Management Department and nursing leaders at St. Mary's Regional Medical Center identified an increase in the fall rate of our patients. The group believed this was primarily occurring on our medical–surgical neurology unit as well as our rehabilitation units. Through the efforts of a multidisciplinary team, specific measures to identify individual unit fall rates and to decrease overall incidents were identified and implemented. These measures included the purchase of new air mattresses to decrease the use of air overlays, new beds each equipped with a bed alarm, and new signage that denoted patients that were at an increased risk of falling. These measures, combined with an increased emphasis on education, have significantly decreased our fall rates and improved the safety of our patients.

NDNQI Startup Consideration

St. Mary's Regional Medical Center began participating in the National Database for Nursing Quality Indicators (NDNQI) in 2002. We began with and continue to use the following indicators: Falls Data, Nursing Care Hours, Patient Days Data, RN Education Data, and Ulcer Data. For St. Mary's, NDNQI was initially used as a means to track our data and to benchmark it on a national level against other hospitals of similar size. Initially, reactions to the information and process were mixed due to the amount of time it took to gather data as well as the lack of familiarity with the benchmarking reports. We knew that this would be a beneficial tool to us; however, it wasn't until the data started to come back that we began to realize the importance of what we were tracking. One major obstacle was learning how to sort through the large volume of data in the

FIGURE 1.
NDNQI Data Reporting and Sharing at St. Mary's

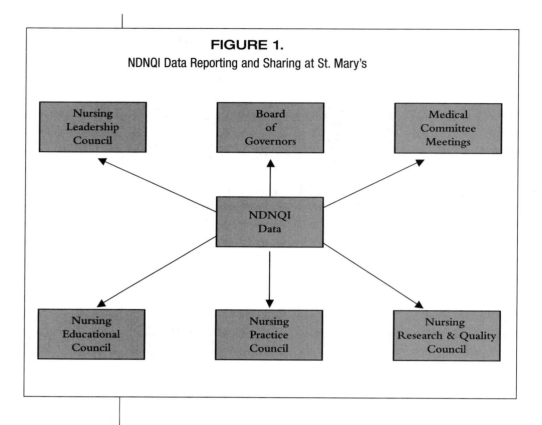

Quality Measurement and Reporting

Quality improvement data are reported at St. Mary's in a variety of ways. The fall data are captured in incident reports which in the past have been a paper format but are now moving to an electronic format. The unit the patient fell on, risk factors, time, date, age, type of fall, and comments to further describe the incident are all captured and tracked in a general report. Data from these reports entered into NDNQI include the unit, the month of occurrence, the age and gender of the patient, whether the fall was assisted, injury level, risk assessment, risk assessment scale, risk assessment score, recency of event, at-risk identification prior to fall, use of physical restraints, and documentation of prior falls. The fall data, along with other nursing indicators, are compiled into a nursing dashboard that is easy to read and quickly identifies upward or downward trending. Our dashboard is a two-page report that gives an overview of quarterly data regarding each of our nursing indicators: length of stay, nursing hours per patient day, overtime, registry/agency nurse hours, nursing staff injury, medication errors, patient falls, falls with injury, decubitus prevention, and percent of patients with hospital-acquired pressure ulcers.

reports and then use it to improve our outcomes. Now we are more familiar with the system, which has helped to make it less time consuming and more useful to us. After five years of participation, we continue to learn more about what the data represent as well as how we can best use it in our decision-making processes. It has been and will continue to be something that we routinely use when we are making both nursing and patient care decisions.

Our NDNQI data and national comparative data are reported regularly at Nursing Research and Quality Council, Nursing Practice Council, Nursing Education Council, Nursing Leadership Council, with the Board of Governors, and at Medical Committee meetings as needed (Figure 1). Sharing the data with each group has increased buy-in and fostered a desire to know how our organization is performing and how we compare with others. The data have helped our organization make important decisions that have improved patient care, in particular, regarding patient falls.

Quality Improvement

In reviewing the inpatient fall data for adjusted patient days, we noted an increase in the rate of patient falls (Figure 2). The data were gathered prior to St. Mary's involvement in NDNQI and represented all inpatient nursing areas.

The quality/risk management department was the first to recognize an overall upward trend in fall rates. Upon identification of the problem, a multidisciplinary team was formed to identify ways to decrease the fall rate. They began by drilling down into the detailed data. The team then initiated the Plan-Do-Check-Act (PDCA) performance improvement method, completed a literature review, established goals, and defined elements of fall prevention.

The first element of the fall improvement plan was an individualized assessment. We needed to ensure that we had consistent initial and ongoing assessments of our patients and that the likelihood of a fall was identified for each patient. Each admission assessment included identification of risk factors and the assessment was reviewed by a registered nurse to determine if the patient had a high risk of falling. If a patient was identified to be at high risk of having a fall, then the fall prevention protocol was established and fall precautions implemented. The essential components of our hospital policy and daily procedures include: documentation of the initial fall risk, teaching both patient and family about fall prevention, and ongoing assessment of fall risk with each shift.

In addition to assessment, the team chose to work on prioritizing outcomes, individualizing the fall risk assessment, and monitoring each patient's specific needs. Intervention with the least restrictive protocol was encouraged. All staff were encouraged to communicate the fall risk as a part of the nurse-to-nurse report and reports to other departments, such as physical medicine. If a patient fell, evaluation of the situation was

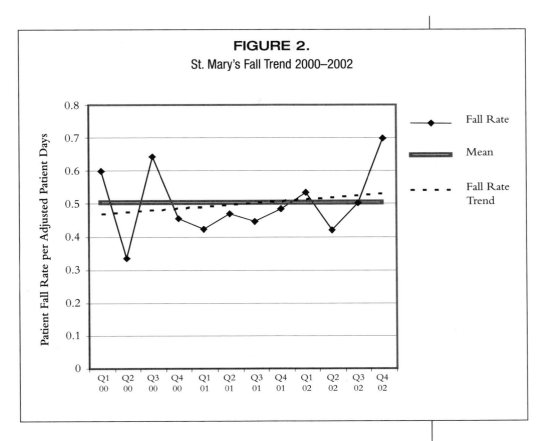

FIGURE 2.
St. Mary's Fall Trend 2000–2002

conducted quickly to determine if other appropriate measures could be implemented.

The new prevention programs included new mattresses with additional comfort and protection for patients. The goal was to decrease the use of air overlays which raised patients higher off the ground than regular mattresses. Other measures included the purchase of new beds for all med–surg and rehabilitation units. The fall team had identified that we were not consistently using bed alarms with our high-risk patients. The new beds were each equipped with their own bed alarm that could be activated easily and were not cumbersome for nursing staff. Finally, new fall risk signs were developed and implemented. Previously, we had used a bright pink laminated sign that stated fall risk. Our staff was becoming very comfortable with the former pink signs and would often comment that they didn't even see the signs. A change was made to colorful, laminated signs that could be changed with each season to add variety

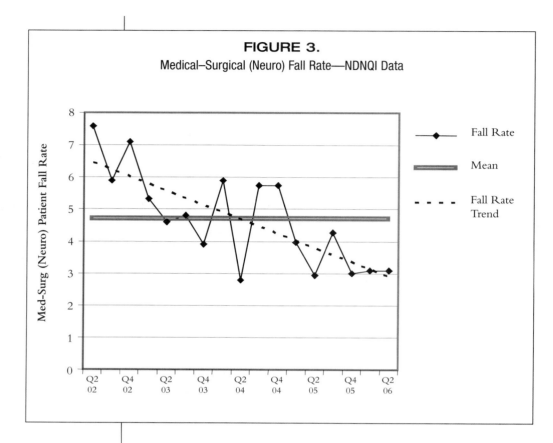

FIGURE 3.
Medical–Surgical (Neuro) Fall Rate—NDNQI Data

Fall Rate

Mean

Fall Rate Trend

Lessons Learned

As with each project, a learning curve was expected, and it took time for all staff to be comfortable with the new measures. To ensure the adoption of our new fall prevention program, we completed education with staff through in-services, discussions at unit meetings, and a hospital-wide "skills day." At this point, staff are now aware of the new measures and all new staff receive information on the new protocol during general hospital orientation. The initial implementation took only about a month, but it has taken the better part of a year for everyone to accept this as part of their routine.

Our new fall prevention program was based on changes in processes and new equipment. No changes were made with nurse staffing levels. Thus, the only costs included the cost of the new mattresses, the cost of the new beds, and the minimal cost of new signs to denote that a patient is at a higher risk of falling. This was a $400,000 capital outlay over the course of three years for a bed replacement plan and mattresses.

and draw the caregiver's eye to the sign. The new signs included falling stars, falling leaves, falling snow, and falling rain. These signs are rotated with the seasons and staff are more aware of patient risk status due to the differences. Another goal with the new signs was that they would catch the attention of the family and friends of the patient to help them realize that this patient was at an increased risk of fall.

Through the six steps of assessment, prioritization, individualization, intervention, communication, and fall evaluation, gaps in the fall program were identified and new systems were implemented. As we have continued to examine the data and implement the new fall assessment process, we have seen an overall decrease trend in our fall rates on both the med–surg (neuro) unit (Figure 3) and the rehabilitation units (Figure 4).

Conclusions and Implications

We have been pleased with the overall decrease in the incidence of falls at St. Mary's. While we have seen a recent drop in our fall rates on these two units, we realize that our work is not done and that it will take continuous monitoring and work toward quality improvement. Participation in NDNQI has been especially beneficial because it has helped us to identify data in a more specific and unit-by-unit basis. Through the continued analysis of our NDNQI data, and comparison to national benchmarks, we will continue to make great strides forward in other areas such as ulcer care and prevention as well as restraint use in all nursing departments. The NDNQI data have provided us evidence on our practice and a means to set some strategic goals such as the achievement of Magnet status. The concrete, data-driven specifics push us to continuously review and improve both our nurse and our patient outcomes, unit-by-unit and within the nursing department as a whole.

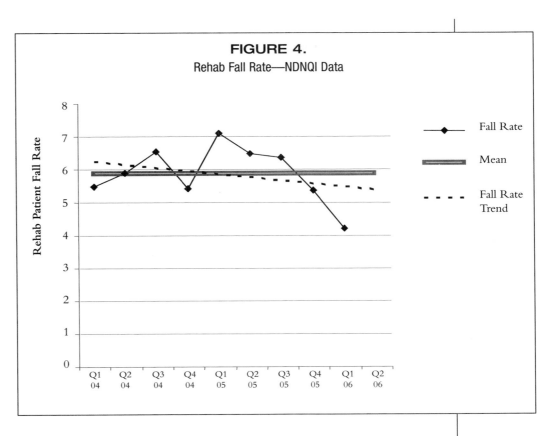

FIGURE 4.
Rehab Fall Rate—NDNQI Data

The authors would also like to acknowledge: Ann Thain, MSW, director of Risk Management; Rita Janousek, RN, director of Medical, Surgical, and RehabCare; Kelley Williams, RN, clinical manager of 2 North, Neurology Medical–Surgical Unit; and Kathy Kerfoot, Quality Manager.

Using NDNQI Data to Monitor the Success of a Unit-Based Falls Prevention Pilot Program

Sue Penque, RN, MSN
Vice President Patient Care
susan.penque@allina.com

Stephanie Cook, RN, MSN
Director Med–Surg Patient Care

Anne Rusch, RN, BSN
Risk Management

United Hospital—St. Paul, Minnesota

Editors' pick:

INSIGHTS & IDEAS FROM THIS FACILITY

Performed audits for protocol compliance and regular rounding for training aided in success.

Facility Summary

Facility	United Hospital—St. Paul, Minnesota www.allina.com
Facility setting	• The geographic area we serve is primarily the east metro area, but we are increasingly seeing patients from Wisconsin, Iowa, North Dakota, and South Dakota. In 2006, we had 28,177 inpatients, 101,196 outpatients, 9845 emergency admissions, 15,976 surgical procedures, and 4,123 births. • John Nasseff Heart Center—122 bed hospital built within United Hospital with level one acute coronary care, same-day recovery unit for open heart surgery. • Bariatric unit on Station 2600—Largest bariatric program in St. Paul. • Geriatric Psychiatric unit—Only geriatric psychiatric unit in St. Paul.
Teaching status	Family practice residency program
Ownership status	Allina Health System
Community demographics	Serving seven Minnesota counties and western Wisconsin
Number of hospital staffed beds	430 staffed beds; 525 total beds. Total :1,237 MNA RNs and 53 LPNs
Indicators used	Falls, Pressure Ulcers, Restraints, Nursing Hours, Certification and Education
System or unit improved	Falls at United Hospital for all patient care areas except OB and Behavioral Health.
Indicator(s) improved	Total fall rate and injury fall rate
QI report card/ document used	Nursing quality indicators
NDNQI participant since	2004
Magnet™ status	The hospital has been engaged in efforts to secure Magnet status since 2002 and applied for Magnet status in 2005.

UNIT PROFILE

Unit size and type	430 staffed beds, 525 total beds
Unit RN staff profile	Usual assignment is 1:4 on days and evenings and 1:5-6 on nights on med–surg and telemetry units.
Unit skill mix of RNs, other personnel	• 7 % RN, 54% AD, 38% BSN, 1% MS/PhD, 10% certification. • Average duration of experience is 11 years.
Organizational structure of unit	The vice president for patient care reports to the president of United Hospital and is a member on the senior management team. The president reports to the CEO of Allina Health System. In addition, the vice president for patient care at United Hospital is a member of the Allina Quality Committee. Directors for patient care at United Hospital report to the vice president for patient care. Units are managed by a nurse manager who has 60 to 110 direct reports.

Using NDNQI Data to Monitor the Success of a Unit-Based Falls Prevention Pilot Program

Sue Penque, RN, MSN
Vice President Patient Care
susan.penque@allina.com

Stephanie Cook, RN, MSN
Director Med–Surg Patient Care

Anne Rusch, RN, BSN
Risk Management

Introduction Summary

United Hospital is a 430-staffed-bed hospital in St. Paul, Minnesota, serving the eastern metropolitan area and western Wisconsin. It is one of several hospitals owned by the Allina Hospitals and Clinics healthcare system. United Hospital participates in local as well as system-wide initiatives with other healthcare facilities owned by Allina. An Allina-wide Falls Group Collaborative helped with reduction of falls throughout the healthcare system.

In early 2002, United Hospital embarked on quality improvement efforts to reduce patient falls in the acute care setting with the goal of achieving zero falls on the medical–surgical patient care units for 2006. An interdisciplinary central falls committee, reporting to the labor management group Nursing Practice Care Delivery, has been accountable for quality improvement efforts that have resulted in a reduction in falls and monitors these on a quarterly basis (Table 1). The numerous resulting interventions achieved since 2002 using NDNQI data include: a new assessment tool used by all nursing staff, improved documentation on flow sheets, review of medications, use of protocols and pathways on "confusion," identification methods for all members of the healthcare team, hourly rounding, assistive personnel for difficult situations, assistive devices for alerting the nursing staff of a high-risk patient, education for all nursing staff, and care plans.

NDNQI Startup Considerations

Prior to 2003, United Hospital was experiencing 10 to 28 falls per month. At that time, measurement was conducted through the quality department and benchmarked within United Hospital. A quality fall reduction team was formed including nursing leadership, nursing staff, pharmacists, risk management, and physicians. The first activity was to review the data from

TABLE 1.

NDNQI Database—Q2-2006

UNIT	National Database of Nursing Quality Indicators (NDNQI) Unit Report: Nurse-Sensitive Indicators—Q2-2006												
	NURSING HOURS				PRESSURE ULCERS		FALLS		INJURY		ASSAULT	
	NHPPD		RN Hours									
	Total # Productive Hours Total # Pt. Days		% Total Nursing Hours Supplied by RNs		Hospital-Acquired (% Patients)		Total Fall Rate per 1,000 Pt. Days		Injury Fall Rate per 1,000 Pt. Days		Physical/Sexual Assaults per 1,000 Pt. Days	
	UH	NDNQI	UH	NDNQI	UH	NDNQI	UH	NDNQI	UH	NDNQI	UH	NDNQI
4400	10.87	8.48	68.10	62.70	n.d.	n.d.	2.77	4.22	0.56	1.24		
4500	10.81	8.35	71.74	62.17	n.d.	n.d.	3.00	3.67	1.20	1.02		
4900	11.52	10.45	74.63	72.08	n.d.	n.d.	0.85	3.39	0.00	0.90		
4920/40	10.97	8.48	74.97	62.70	n.d.	n.d.	1.75	4.22	0.00	1.24		
6900/40	14.43	8.93	65.82	62.97	n.d.	n.d.	1.45	2.89	0.00	0.81		
7900/20	9.93	8.35	68.18	62.17	n.d.	n.d.	4.54	3.67	0.58	1.02		
8900	9.42	8.39	45.34	49.69	n.d.	n.d.	n.d		n.d.		3.09	0.59

all patient care units and compare to the national data reported in the literature as well as identify interventions cited as successful for acute care. All data were reviewed related to severity, time of day, types of interventions being used, medications patients received prior to the fall, location of the patient, clinical diagnosis, and other demographics.

The findings revealed the lack of a consistent assessment tool to identify patients at risk and a wide range of interventions used without an examination of the outcome to the patient. While the majority of falls occurred on the medical surgical units, 50% also occurred in the intensive care, obstetrical units, and behavioral health. The following needs emerged:

- Consistent fall risk tool to be utilized by all nursing staff

- Consistent interventions on all nursing units with individualization for patient populations

- Centralized fall reduction team to provide quality oversight for the hospital

- Alternative devices to reduce falls

- Consistent measurement and definitions

Quality Measurement and Reporting

Based on this information, United Hospital enrolled in NDNQI in 2003 and the medical unit (Unit 4400) became the pilot for strategies to reduce falls at the hospital. The program focused on enhanced observation and the use of visual cues to identify patients at risk for falls. All patients were required to have a fall risk assessment completed each shift and documented on the flow sheet. Education was provided to patients and families on how to avoid falls. A brochure, Ten Tips for Patients, that discusses the patient's role in preventing falls in the hospital, was created by the orthopedics unit

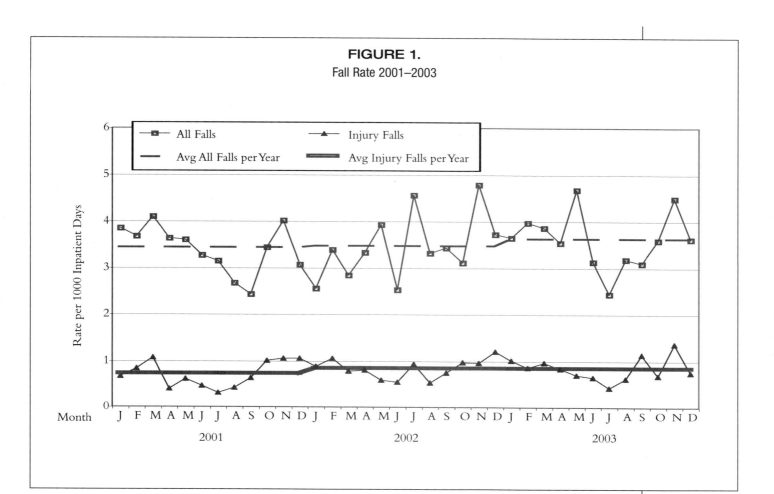

FIGURE 1.
Fall Rate 2001–2003

and implemented at first at United Hospital and later Allina-wide. In summary, the plan included:

- Clear identification of patients at risk for falls to all members of the health team

- Attaching an alarm system to the patient to indicate movement that could cause harm

- Ongoing assessment of the risk

- Review of medications with the physician and pharmacist

- Use of one-to-one attendant, if needed

United Hospital used NDNQI for consistent definitions and benchmarking by incorporating the findings into a hospital-wide nursing quality improvement plan. The benefits of comparing ourselves to other hospitals nationwide far outweighed the benefits of internal benchmarking. Literature reviews were helpful but did not provide current comparison data.

Quality Improvement

The falls reduction program is a continuous process improvement at United Hospital. The key to success is ownership of the initiative by the staff nurses and ongoing support from nursing leadership to review data, educate staff, and monitor and celebrate success. While injury fall rates decreased in 2003, the overall rate of patient falls fluctuated (Figure 1). These results made

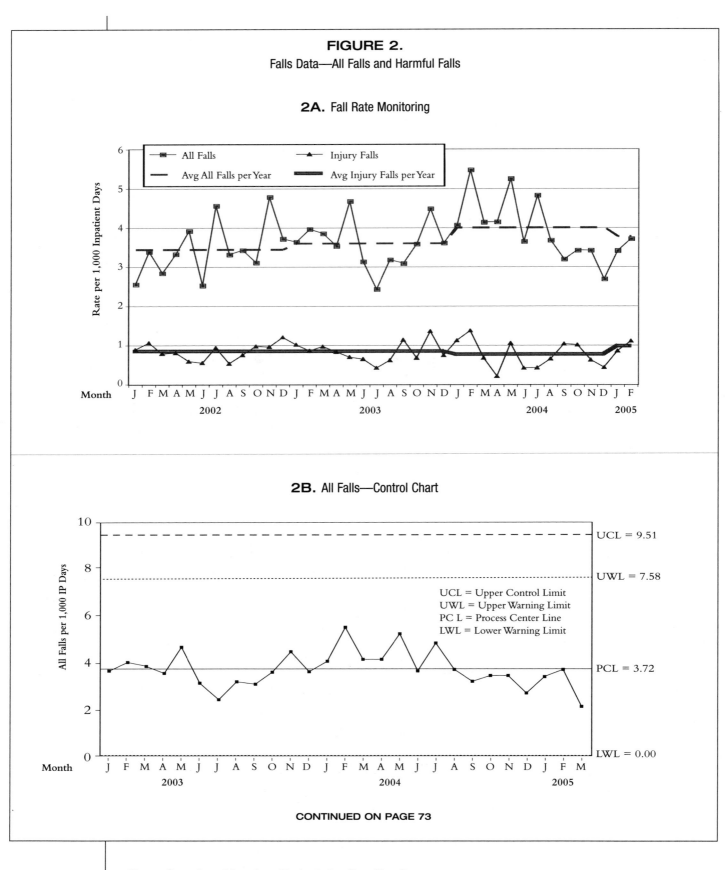

FIGURE 2.
Falls Data—All Falls and Harmful Falls

2A. Fall Rate Monitoring

2B. All Falls—Control Chart

UCL = Upper Control Limit
UWL = Upper Warning Limit
PC L = Process Center Line
LWL = Lower Warning Limit

CONTINUED ON PAGE 73

Transforming Nursing Data Into Quality Care:
Profiles of Quality Improvement in U.S. Healthcare Facilities

FIGURE 2.
Continued

2C. Injury Falls Control Chart

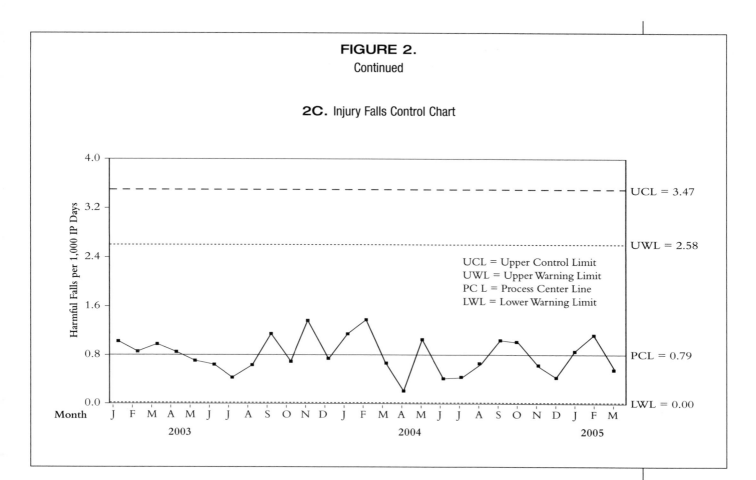

clear that prevention interventions alone without sound means of predicting fall risk do not constitute a complete and accurate approach to improving safety. (Cook, et al. 2004)

United Hospital continued with its quality improvement program and implemented the use of the Ann Hendrich II fall risk assessment tool on all nursing units. Because of the mass implementation and need for further education, fall risk liaisons were identified—nurses who became experts in use of the tool and intervention strategies. These liaisons attended a workshop by Ann Hendrich and were required to attend monthly meetings to help with quality plans. It became the responsibility of the nursing leaders to implement the program on their unit with assistance from the central team at United Hospital. Once patients were identified

as at risk for falls, a magnet indicating "fall risk" was used, along with yellow wrist bands. These visual clues were valued by the healthcare team as a mechanism to quickly identify who was at risk. In addition, nursing assistants were educated to make regular rounds to ensure a safe environment for the patient. One-to-one attendants were used for certain types of patients, when needed. Based on this phase of the program, the overall and harmful fall rates declined (Figure 2).

NDNQI was incorporated into the nursing quality plan for 2005 and 2006. All nursing units at United Hospital were given a score with targets to reduce falls. The Nursing Practice Committee, the hospital's labor management committee with MNA (Minnesota Nurses Association), included reduction of falls as a main initiative. The goal to reduce harmful falls contin-

TABLE 2.
Timeline to Success

2002 **Champions for patient safety set goal to decrease patient falls by 50%.**

United Hospital fall prevention team focus on interventions and institute a fall program. The trigger for interventions was the fall risk score (current tool) or a history of falling prior to admission. These indicators are available to staff. Identified need for research-based tool.

Tab alarms pilot on medicine.

Determine and obtain visual cues for fall interventions (stickers, arm bands, magnet).

2003 **Goal for 2003 is to reduce falls that cause harm by 50%.**

Allina Fall Group, including United Hospital, compares Schmid Fall Risk Assessment Tool, Morse Fall Scale, Hendrich Fall Risk Model, Conley Scale. Factors = time to complete, levels of risk, inter-rater reliability, sensitivity, specificity. United Hospital pilots Hendrich Model.

Pilot of Hendrich II starts, excluding BHS, ICU, and birth center. Fall rates in birth center and ICU were low at that time and therefore were excluded in the beginning.

Memo to all nursing staff with fall rate data and congratulations for great work. Reminder to continue to focus on scoring with the Hendrich Model.

2004 **United Hospital enrolls in NDNQI to establish common measurements and benchmarking.**

Fall model is part of Competency Day for nursing staff and PCAs.

Confirmation from Ann Hendrich regarding: attendance at Allina Falls Collaborative to be held at United Hospital in March. Message to sites to assemble teams to represent their hospitals and to be able to assist with implementation of the model.

Allina Falls Collaborative held at United Hospital.

Plan put forth for system-wide implementation of Hendrich model at United Hospital. Liaisons to assist with implementation. United Hospital seen as flagship for Allina on fall prevention.

Toileting rounds on medicine unit decrease the fall rate by 50%. Nurse or aide offers to assist patient to the bathroom every other hour while the patient is awake.

2005 **Allina wide goal established for reduction of falls in all areas.**

Geriatric Psych unit enrolled in program with major reduction in overall falls. Continued focus on reduction of falls

2006 **United Hospital participates in IHI fall reduction program.**

Medicine Telemetry pilots quality improvement program focusing on rounds

ued but the overall rate continued to be higher than the plan. After examining the reasons why program progress seemed to be stagnant, it was found that without ongoing monitoring of the plan of care, nursing staff were not focused on the goal. To achieve the goals, a goal to reduce overall falls was added to the evaluation process for all leaders within United Hospital. This created renewed interest and investment in the plans.

Lessons Learned

Falls were significantly reduced at United Hospital due to vigilant monitoring of the interventions, fall risk scores, and outcomes achieved. On a quarterly basis, the Nursing Practice Committee reviews the NDNQI data and makes recommendations for improvement. Audits are randomly done to ensure the assessment tool is used by 100% of nursing staff. In the near future, an electronic record will aid in completion of this tool by all staff and serve as another mechanism to communicate about those patients at risk.

Conclusions and Implications

However, such quality improvement work is never done. The goal would be to achieve zero falls on all units. Further review of the literature suggests that regular rounding on patients, scheduled bathroom visits, ambulating patients at regular intervals, use of family members in care of patients, and ongoing education of the patient and family are critical factors to success. Several of the medicine units have implemented these interventions and have achieved zero falls over several months.

A summary of activity is included for review (Table 2). Overall, there were no barriers to implementing this plan and the costs only included staff and leadership time which involved approximately $60,000 in educational training over a one-year period. The key to these successes stems from nurses acknowledging their role in achieving better outcomes and celebrating success. The use of nursing research and an established national database were crucial for the program. Thanks to nursing leadership from advanced practice roles, nursing management and staff, fall reduction goals are being achieved on all units at United Hospital.

References

Cook S, et al. Preventing falls: A hospital intervention program assesses risk. *Minnesota Physician* 2004; July: 28–29.

Hendrich AL, et al. Validation of the Hendrich II fall risk model: A large concurrent case/control study of hospitalized patients *Appl Nurs Res* 2003; 16(1): 9–21. [Corrected published erratum appears in *Appl Nurs Res* 2003; 16(3): 208.]

Holmes P. Supporting older people: Promoting falls prevention. *Brit J Comm Nurs* 2006; 11(6): 247–8,250.

QuickStats from the national center for health statistics. Annual rate of nonfatal, medically attended fall injuries among adults aged greater than or equal to 65 years— United States, 2001–2003. *MMWR* 2006;55(31):857.

Whitehead CH, et al. Attitudes to falls and injury prevention: What are the barriers to implementing falls prevention strategies? *Clin Rehab* 2006; 20(6): 536–542.

Pressure Ulcer Prevalence

Defined:

A pressure ulcer is any lesion caused by **unrelieved pressure** resulting in damage of underlying tissue. They may be located over bony prominences or skin surfaces subject to excess pressure such as under a medical device/equipment. They are staged according to the extent of observable tissue damage. The nurse observer should be able to distinguish a pressure ulcer from other types of wounds and skin conditions (e.g., venous or arterial ulcers, diabetic foot ulcers, yeast infections, maceration, perineal dermatitis, skin tears, or operating room-acquired cautery burns). Count the number of pressure ulcers on each patient, whether acquired since admission to your facility or acquired before admission.

Hospital acquired refers to new ulcer(s) developed **after** admission to a facility. Also termed nosocomial or facility-acquired. The hospital admission assessment should be reviewed for the presence of ulcers. If there is no documentation that the ulcer was present on admission, then the ulcer(s) should be counted as hospital acquired.

Formulas:

Total Pressure Ulcer Prevalence: Prevalence Number of patients with Ulcers/ Number of patients in survey

Hospital Acquired Pressure Ulcer: Prevalence Number of patients with Hospital Acquired Ulcers / Number of patient in survey

Graphing NDNQI Trend Data on the Intranet Supports Zero Tolerance of Hospital Acquired Pressure Ulcers

Kathleen Johnson, MSN, RN, CNA
Nurse Manager, MICU
Christiana Hospital
katjohnson@christianacare.org

Joanne Bramble, RN, CPHQ
Administrative Associate, Performance Improvement
Christiana Hospital

Denise Netta-Turner, BSN, RN, CWON
Wound, Ostomy, Continence Nurse
Wilmington Hospital

Christiana Care Health System—Wilmington, Delaware

Editors' pick:

INSIGHTS & IDEAS FROM THIS FACILITY

Specialists (wound/ostomy continence) made the difference when assigned to specific units to help involve all staff.

Facility Summary

Facility	Christiana Care Health System—Wilmington, Delaware www.Christianacare.org
Facility setting	CCHS is a regional center known for excellence in cardiology, cancer, and women's health services, as well as a Level 1 trauma care and Level 3 neonatal intensive care (both the highest intensity levels). CCHS operates two hospitals, transitional care services, preventive medicine and rehabilitation services, a network of primary care physician offices, and offers an extensive range of outpatient and home health services.
Teaching status	University-affiliated teaching hospital (Thomas Jefferson University Medical College)
Ownership status	Private, nonprofit healthcare system
Community demographics	CCHS provides services in a market composed of 1.2 million individuals in Delaware and adjacent counties in Pennsylvania, Maryland, and New Jersey. Over 518,000 of these live in CCHS's primary market of New Castle County, Delaware. Over the next five years, the population is expected to grow by 1.5 % in New Castle County and 2.1% in adjacent communities. The median age of the population in New Castle County is 42, with 12% over age 65. Median household income is $46,148. Approximately 12% of the population is uninsured.
Number of hospital staffed beds	1,071 beds in two hospitals
Indicators used	Hospital acquired pressure ulcers
System or unit improved	Both system-wide (CCHS) and unit-specific (MICU)
Indicator(s) improved	Hospital acquired pressure ulcers
QI report card/ document used	NDNQI
NDNQI participant since	2002
Magnet™ status	Applying

UNIT PROFILE

Unit size and type	Medical Intensive Care Unit: 12 beds
Unit RN staff profile	40 to 45 RNs; 40% > 10 years in ICU; 20% > 25 years at CCHS
Skill mix of RNs, other personnel	100% RN staff
Organizational structure of unit	Shared decision-making model

Graphing NDNQI Trend Data on the Intranet Supports Zero Tolerance of Hospital Acquired Pressure Ulcers

Kathleen Johnson, MSN, RN, CNA
Nurse Manager, MICU
katjohnson@christianacare.org

Joanne Bramble, RN, CPHQ
Administrative Associate, Performance Improvement

Denise Netta-Turner, BSN, RN, CWON
Wound, Ostomy, Continence Nurse
Wilmington Hospital

Introductory Summary: The Initial MICU Situation

The Medical Intensive Care Unit (MICU) at Christiana Hospital, part of the Christiana Care Health System (CCHS), has exhibited a hospital-acquired pressure ulcers (HAPU) prevalence rate below the NDNQI mean for critical care units over the past five quarters (Q1-2005–Q1-2006). Before this accomplishment, MICU demonstrated one of the highest prevalence rates among all of the Christiana Hospital nursing units. MICU's success story is one that articulates and embraces a complex challenge, called for changing nursing culture and practice, and required a collaborative effort among all the nursing departments. A hospital-wide interdisciplinary team formed out of the project to define a standard goal of zero tolerance for hospital-acquired skin breakdown. Starting in 2002, National Database of Nursing Quality Indicators (NDNQI) data was utilized to trend progress and benchmark CCHS units against similar units nationally. Among the results were that the CCHS point prevalence rate for HAPUs stabilized at nearly half what they had been two years before and the MICU rate dropped to zero from almost 42% in less than two years.

Facility At A Glance

Christiana Care Health System is one of the largest healthcare providers in the Mid-Atlantic region. CCHS has a Level I Trauma Center and teaching hospital serving Delaware and parts of Pennsylvania, Maryland, and New Jersey. CCHS provides services in multiple settings that include two acute care facilities: Christiana Hospital, a 780-bed facility in suburban Newark, Delaware; Wilmington Hospital, a 291-bed facility in the center of the city of Wilmington; and one post-acute care facility, Riverside Transitional Care, a 108-bed facility that specializes in care of complex wounds. Outpatient wound care services are also provided by the Wound Care Center at the Riverside campus, offering interdisciplinary and comprehensive wound care for patients with chronic non-healing wounds. The Christiana Care Visiting Nurse Association offers home care for those in need throughout Delaware.

The MICU is a 12-bed intensive care unit at Christiana Hospital with an average daily census of 11.2 critically ill, multisystem-failure patients. The staff is composed of 40 to 45 RNs. There is strong staff leadership in the unit of 11 fully functioning committees, including a performance improvement (PI) committee with a dedication to evidence-based practice, patient advocacy, and professional pride in quality patient care and positive clinical outcomes. Forty percent of the staff RNs have been working in the ICU for more than 10 years and 20% have worked at CCHS longer than 25 years. Staff mentors include a staff development specialist and clinical nurse specialist as well as a variety of other hospital specialists available for consultation.

The CCHS department of nursing supports a shared decision-making structure that is lateral, augments communication, and includes professional nursing representation in all levels of decision-making. This structure consists of four system-level councils for: evidence-based nursing practice, education, quality and safety, and professional nursing. Unit-level councils align with the purposes and goals of the system councils. The integrity of this decision-making model relies upon meaningful participation of professional staff nurses. The model empowers the professional nursing staff to contribute collectively to the deci-

sion-making process related to nursing practice, quality, and competence.

NDNQI Startup Considerations

For many years, CCHS collected internal data reflecting unit performance of patient outcomes. The department of nursing attempted to identify indicators that were reflective of nursing practices. In the attempt to measure and determine improvement, CCHS was unable to validate real progress compared to other organizations. Literature searches of nursing journals and other publications failed to provide comparative data at either a national or an individual institutional level. This was the result of a lack of both standardized indicator definitions and consistent methods to collect, calculate, and report outcomes.

In seeking out other facilities recognized for nursing excellence, the department of nursing discovered the existence of the NDNQI program. By joining this initiative, CCHS nursing hoped to provide a mechanism to assess nursing practice outcomes and achieve performances at a level of excellence. For the first time, benchmarking data by same unit type and hospital size gave each unit a realistic assessment of their practice performance and possibly a goal to strive for. In addition, the NDNQI database collected data from hospitals on the nursing hours of care and the staffing mix. This information could be valuable in tracking and trending for potential correlation to any of the nurse-sensitive indicators of care.

Initially, many staff were unfamiliar with and resistant to the very new concept of nurse-sensitive indicators. Education and re-education were required to raise the level of understanding and achieve buy-in. Once the nurses could see the positive impact in patient outcomes, the NDNQI standards became accepted CCHS-wide.

HAPU Quality Improvement: Initial Steps

The CCHS skin team was formed with interdisciplinary membership from across the system to reduce the prevalence of HAPU. The team was led by a wound ostomy continence (WOC) nurse and a physician gerontologist and included:

- Infection control physician
- WOC nurses
- Direct care nurses
- Gerontology clinical nurse specialists
- Nurse managers
- Staff development specialists
- Geriatric clinical pharmacist
- Dietician
- Physical therapist
- Visiting nurse
- Wound Care Center director
- Performance improvement data analysts

Utilizing the Plan-Do-Check-Act (PDCA) model for performance improvement, the team began evaluating current practice. The NDNQI data were reviewed for the HAPU indicator to determine unit performance compared to the national mean by unit type and hospital size. An extensive literature search ensued for evidence-based practice. The team then developed a care management guideline (CMG) that would provide standards for skin care throughout CCHS.

For the MICU nurses, as well as many other nurses on inpatient nursing units, the nursing care standard included turning patients every two hours and keeping them clean and dry. All nurses believed they accomplished care per the standard with efficiency and obtained the most reasonably expected outcomes. The sentiment at the time was that the MICU had the really sick, chronically ill, malnourished, unstable patients who were always at the highest risk of acquiring skin pressure breakdown. In short, the MICU's working assumption was, "Skin breakdown was inevitable." Practice changes that could improve outcomes in HAPUs were not thought to be possible with the MICU patient population. These ICU nurses, who were expert in critical care, were thought to be providing the best evidence-based practice to save skin integrity.

In addition, the nurses were reluctant to take ownership for their unit's HAPU prevalence rates, because they felt the skin breakdown often occurred on another unit prior to the patient being transferred to them.

Initially, the HAPU education program was developed using a train-the-trainer model, including representatives from all units. MICU, like all the other units, selected direct care nurses as trainers. They attended in-services on staging of wounds and differentiation of causes of skin breakdown (i.e., fungal, pressure, irritants, shearing). After the initial education of the staff nurses and the patient care technicians, education was integrated into other ongoing educational programs, as appropriate, such as nursing orientation, We Improve Senior Health (WISH), patient care technicians training, nurse internship programs, and a wound care workshop.

Education was also disseminated to the units through the department of nursing performance improvement (PI) council. Representatives from each unit learned how to use the CCHS data collection tool and monitored skin breakdown routinely. They learned about the NDNQI database and how to read and interpret the NDNQI reports. The MICU's PI chairperson had exposure to the hospital-wide efforts and was aware that the suggested practice changes were supported by evidence in the literature. She brought new energy and challenge to the MICU PI committee. It was her commitment and drive that convinced the MICU team that they needed to look at an old problem with new vision. Skin breakdown, not unlike ventilator-associated pneumonia, was no longer considered inevitable in the MICU.

"Zero tolerance" for hospital-acquired pressure ulcers was becoming the mantra for patient care in the MICU. Because patients frequently move from one unit to another as their care needs change, it took an entire healthcare system working as a team to achieve this goal. With prevention as the key, the nursing staff have become more accountable in taking ownership of unit-based care by increasing vigilance and becoming proactive to improve skin outcomes. MICU's participation, with all nursing units, has engaged staff in setting their goal of zero tolerance for HAPU. Activities included improving documentation tools, making resource information easily accessible, providing educational opportunities, becoming a key voice in selection of support surfaces, selecting additional wound care products, and participating in a WOC-sponsored research project that is comparing products to prevent skin breakdown.

The initial learning curve required determining just what the data meant, not only to each unit, but to the whole healthcare system. Unlike unit-specific data on patient falls, skin prevalence data presented a greater challenge in that the nursing team on any given unit could not solely impact their prevalence rates. The response for unit prevalence rates for high HAPU were that "it didn't happen on this unit—not on my watch!" As the skin prevalence data were presented and analyzed each quarter, and multiple units reported rates above the "mean," CCHS soon came to realize that the problem was not fixable by addressing units individually. A system-wide approach was needed because patients often needed multiple transfers across units to provide the needed level of care.

HAPU Quality Improvement: Further Implementation

Using the PDCA model, CCHS staff were able to prevent and decrease the prevalence of HAPUs through improvement of assessments, documentation, and treatment of skin impairment.

As previously stated, NDNQI was selected as the database that would be used to measure and report the nurse-sensitive indicators, providing a quarterly comparison by unit type and by hospital size. Because CCHS is committed to providing excellence in care, data on the prevalence of skin impairment are collected on a monthly basis. CCHS established a comprehensive database for each unit. This included NDNQI data showing trends over time for the presence of hospital-acquired pressure ulcers.

In addition to the indicators defined by the NDNQI, CCHS nursing also decided to collect and trend data on the use of specialty beds, length of stay, and location/site of HAPUs, as well as perform focused monitoring on the use of in-dwelling Foley catheters and the criteria for their use. Of course, "data are only data" unless they can be accurately interpreted and used to support improvement in systems, knowledge, and performance. The CCHS intranet provides a central location and forum for the department of nursing to access their information on performance improvement data.

In 2004, a web site—Performance Improvement and JCAHO Readiness—was developed by the data acquisition and management department, in conjunction with the department of nursing, to display unit outcomes of quality service to CCHS patients. Access and orientation to the use of this web site was and continues to be provided to unit-based nursing performance improvement chairs, unit-based clinical nurse specialists, and all levels of those in nursing leadership.

Data that are shared on this web site include: care management guidelines, which contain algorithms and pathways for patient care; staffing effectiveness reports; patient satisfaction reports; and restraint management results.

Written reports from NDNQI are received and distributed quarterly to all participating unit-based performance improvement chairs and nursing leadership. The results are also displayed graphically for the patient falls and hospital-acquired pressure ulcers indicators on this web site to help nurses easily assess their unit's quarterly performance. Results are also supplied by service and by facility each quarter.

The graphs can be printed easily and displayed for the entire nursing staff on the performance improvement bulletin boards located in the nursing lounge of each participating nursing unit. All direct care nurses can utilize their outcome data to develop and monitor action plans to improve patient care.

In Q4-2003, CCHS had a HAPU point prevalence of 6.31% steadily reducing to 3.04% for Q2-2006 (Figure 1). The trend line is a simple linear trend reflecting an overall 50% decline in the hospital's HAPU prevalence. This decline was steady and averaged 5% per quarter. In addition, 23 out of 25 nursing units were below the NDNQI mean for HAPUs for Q2-2006.

MICU, with a capacity of 12 patients, had the highest point prevalence rate for HAPUs in Q4-04 of 42.86%. The NDNQI mean for critical care units was 15.32%. In the next five quarters (Q1-2005–Q1-2006), MICU has maintained a point prevalence of 0% (Figure 2).

Lessons Learned

For data to be useful, they must be available to nursing staff in a form that is easy to interpret and identify

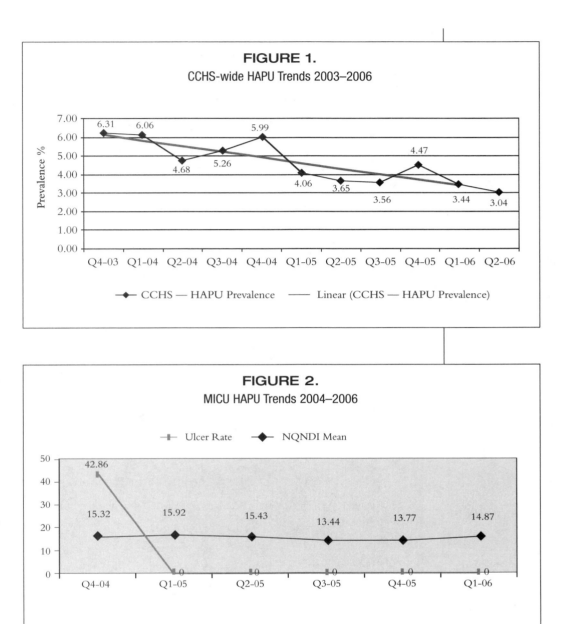

FIGURE 1.
CCHS-wide HAPU Trends 2003–2006

FIGURE 2.
MICU HAPU Trends 2004–2006

trends. This transforms data into information that nursing staff can analyze and use to make appropriate improvement in systems, knowledge, and performance. CCHS developed a mechanism to meet this need in relation to NDNQI data by creating a designated web site on our internal intranet system dedicated to the display of NDNQI data. The nursing management team and the staff can view their data in colored graphic format that is easily understood. The graphs are developed in both line and bar graph format. The line

Once the Planning Is Done:
PDCA in Action at Christiana Hospital's MICU

During the planning phase, the MICU team reviews the data and the current care processes for patients at risk for skin impairment. The prevention itself happens during the next three PDCA phases— Do, Check, Act.

The "Do" Phase

In this phase, the skin team implemented the following strategies:

- Revised the system-wide skin integrity care management guideline (CMG) to reflect best practice.

- Increased the effectiveness and efficiency of wound ostomy continence (WOC) nurses by assigning them to specific patient care units. This resulted in more timely consultations, provided continuity in patient care, and built a team rapport with the unit staff.

- Formed interdisciplinary unit teams to perform weekly skin rounds for early identification of patients at risk for skin impairment and to assure implementation of preventive measures.

- Introduced more effective wound care products.

- Implemented knitted cotton bed sheets to provide a softer surface and eliminate shrinkage.

- Evaluated the use of gel surfaces and obtained improved products for use in the operating rooms for positioning of patients.

- Revised the CCU flow sheet for documenting skin assessment and plan of care to provide trending of improvement in skin impairment by location of breakdown (Figure 3).

- Developed three different wound care order sets.

- Initiated a WOC nurse-led research project to better manage patients with fecal incontinence to prevent skin impairment.

- Improved the process for obtaining vacuum assisted closure (VAC) therapy:

  - Kept pumps on-site to initiate treatment in a timely fashion

  - Developed a clinical practice guideline for VAC therapy

  - Incorporated VAC therapy application and management into critical skills competencies for staff

- Developed a skin documentation tool for the emergency departments to record an assessment of skin breakdown on admission (Figure 4).

continued on next page

Transforming Nursing Data Into Quality Care:
Profiles of Quality Improvement in U.S. Healthcare Facilities

- Revised the post skin impairment analysis tool for completion when skin breakdown identified to provide information for analysis and data for trending.

- Provided physician education regarding:

  - Skin integrity CMG

  - New wound care products

  - Specialty bed surfaces available

- Developed a web site on the CCHS intranet for skin care references :

  - Tool for identifying location of wounds

  - "For Your Information" patient education sheet for interventions to prevent skin breakdown

  - Skin product information

  - Guide for selection of wound care products by stage of wound

- Evaluated specialty beds and surfaces and worked with vendors to develop improved products to assure patient safety.

The "Check" Phase

Plotting and evaluating of NDNQI data were ongoing. A downward trend line for HAPU was identified across both hospitals. The MICU's data showed significant improvement, which is reflective of the collaborative efforts system-wide in preventing and reducing hospital-acquired pressure ulcers.

The "Act" Phase

The goal was to continue improving maintenance of skin integrity through a team effort and ongoing education. Lessons learned during this process include:

- Everyone in the organization must have the same goals regarding skin breakdown.

- Everyone must be able to track skin breakdown from admission to discharge.

- Everyone must be able to differentiate pressure breakdown from other causes (i.e., shearing, fungal).

- Everyone must take action quickly when the risk of breakdown increases (loss of mobility, hypotension, and malnourishment) or a patient's skin is getting red (Stage I).

- Every nursing unit needs a "champion" to empower their own staff.

• • •

CHRISTIANA CARE
HEALTH SERVICES

PRESSURE ULCER RECORD AND PLAN OF CARE

Instructions for use:
1. Complete on a 3 day basis after pressure ulcer is identified or with changes in ulcer.
2. Complete one record per wound site.

Site of Wound: _____ **# of forms used:** _____

Date WOC Nurse consulted _____ (Wound Ostomy Continence)   side 1

PRESSURE ULCER STAGES			
I	Non-blanchable erythema of intact skin; The precursor to cell death/skin ulceration. Discoloration of the skin, warmth, edema or induration may be indicators in individuals with darker pigmented skin.	III	Full thickness of skin is lost, involving damage or necrosis of subcutaneous tissues, which may extend down to but not through underlying fascia; deep crater with or without undermining adjacent tissue.
II	Partial thickness skin loss involving epidermis and / or dermis. The ulcer is superficial and presents clinically as an abrasion, blister or shallow crater.	IV	A full thickness of skin loss with extensive destruction, tissue necrosis, or damage to muscle, bone, or supporting structures (such as tendon and joint capsule); deep crater with or without undermining of adjacent tissue; may have exposed bone or muscle.

(   ) Wound unstageable

Date	Stage	Length(cm) head to toe	Width (cm) hip to hip	Depth (cm)	Color	Tunneling (cm/o'clock)	Undermining (cm/o'clock)	Drainage (type/amount)	Odor (yes/no)	Treatment / Intervention	WOC Nurse Visit	Initials

Key:
Nonstageable: wounds covered with non-viable tissue such as eschar. Deep purple discoloration of wounds may indicate deeper tissue damage.
Key for color code for wounds: a. red = granulation tissue; b. pink = clear, smooth wound base; c. yellow = slough; d. black = eschar, leather-like appearance; e. other = any other color
Key for Secretions/Drainage: Y = yellow; TAN = tan; W = white; B = brown; GR = green; FR = frothy; BL = bloody; PK = pink; sm = small ; MOD = moderate; LG = large; ser = serosanguineous; TH = thick; cl = clear

Initials	Signature/Title	Print Name	Initials	Signature/Title	Print Name

21673 S(   )(0705)C   PLAN OF CARE - Pressure

(3) Hole 1/4 1 3/8 c-to-c

reflects a trend line over quarters and the bar graph is a composite of all of the units participating in the NDNQI database. Those 'below the mean" fall into the RED section of the bar and those "above the mean" are in the green section of the bar. It is each unit's goal to be in the green. The NDNQI data graphs are printed by unit, so that they could be reviewed by the unit-based performance improvement teams, presented at the unit staff meetings, and also be displayed on the performance improvement section of the unit bulletin

FIGURE 3.

Continued

PRESSURE ULCER RECORD AND PLAN OF CARE
Side 2

Treatments/Interventions

A. Moisture Barrier
    1. A & D Ointment
    2. No Sting Barrier
    3. Secura Dimethicone Protectant
    4. Zinc Oxide 20%
    5. Zinc Oxide 40%
    6. Zinc Oxide and Stomahesive Powder Mixture
    8. Other

B. Moisturizer
    1. Formula II
    2. Secura Dimethicone Protectant
    3. Other

C. Healing Ointment-Xenoderm

D. Topical Antifungal
    1. Nystatin Cream
    2. Nystatin Ointment
    3. Nystatin Powder
    4. Other

E. Topical Antimicrobial
    1. Bacitracin
    2. Bactroban
    3. Silvadene Cream
    4. Other

F. Wound Dressing
    1. Foam
    2. Hydrocolloid
    3. Hydrofiber
    4. Hydrogel-Amorphous
    5. Hydrogel-Sheet
    6. Impregnated Dressing
    7. Transparent Film
    8. Wet-Moist
    9. Wound Emulsion
    10. Other

G. Topical Enzymatic Debrider
    1. Accuzyme
    2. Panafil
    3. Santyl
    4. Other

H. Secondary Dressing
    1. Dry Gauze
    2. Foam
    3. Kerlix
    4. Moist Gauze
    5. Transparent Film
    6. Other

I. Negative Pressure Wound Therapy (VAC - Vacuum Assisted Closure)

Specialty Bed Codes for Treatment/Intervention.

AC-O	Acucair Overlay
B	Bariatric (with foam mattress)
CL	Clinitron
CLR	Clinitron Rite Hite
E	Flexicair Eclipse Mattress (replacement)
FL	Flexicair Bed
G	Gaymar Overlay
MA	Bariatric (w/ Mighty Air mattress)
MC3	Flexicair MC3 (w/ scales)
H	Hill-Rom Low Bed w/ pressure relieving mattress
NU	Neuropedic Mattress
OP	Optimal Specialty Mattress
S	Total Care Sport (pulmonary bed)
ST	Stryker Low Bed w/ pressure relieving mattress
TC	Total Care/ICU Bed

Pressure Ulcer Sites in the Pelvic Region

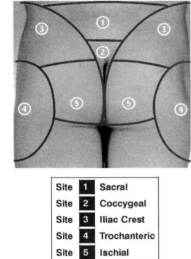

Site	1	Sacral
Site	2	Coccygeal
Site	3	Iliac Crest
Site	4	Trochanteric
Site	5	Ischial

board in each staff lounge.

The MICU unit performance improvement committee and the management team identified an opportunity for improvement for reduction in HAPU prevalence. Their data indicated the need to redesign a process using a systematic approach with the PDCA model for performance improvement. In the planning phase, the team reviewed the data and the current care processes for identifying and managing patients at risk

FIGURE 4.

Documentation Tool for Skin Breakdown Assessment at Admission

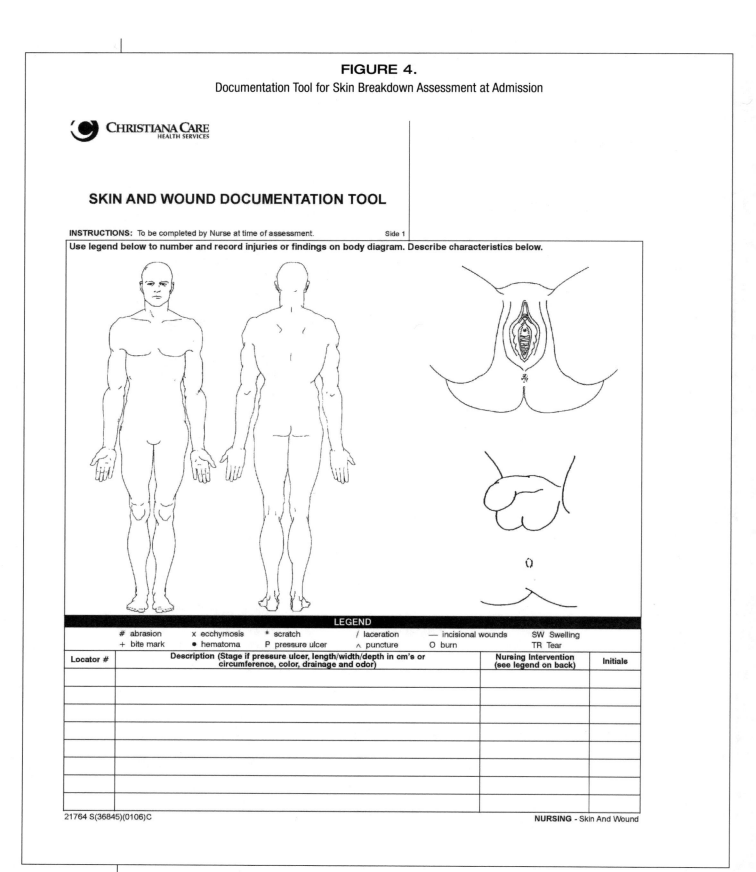

CHRISTIANA CARE
HEALTH SERVICES

SKIN AND WOUND DOCUMENTATION TOOL

INSTRUCTIONS: To be completed by Nurse at time of assessment.   Side 1

Use legend below to number and record injuries or findings on body diagram. Describe characteristics below.

LEGEND					
# abrasion	x ecchymosis	* scratch	/ laceration	— incisional wounds	SW Swelling
+ bite mark	● hematoma	P pressure ulcer	∧ puncture	O burn	TR Tear

Locator #	Description (Stage if pressure ulcer, length/width/depth in cm's or circumference, color, drainage and odor)	Nursing Intervention (see legend on back)	Initials

21764 S(36845)(0106)C

NURSING - Skin And Wound

Transforming Nursing Data Into Quality Care:
Profiles of Quality Improvement in U.S. Healthcare Facilities

FIGURE 4.
Continued

CHRISTIANA CARE
HEALTH SERVICES

SKIN AND WOUND DOCUMENTATION TOOL

Side 2

Locator #	Description (Stage if pressure ulcer, length/width/depth in cm's or circumference, color, drainage and odor)	Nursing Intervention	Initials

Nursing Interventions Legend

(A) Initiate turning and repositioning on a 2 hour basis; elevate heels off bed and pad elbow with Tegaderm
(B) Specialty bed ordered
(C) Consult Wound Ostomy Continence Nurse (stage III or greater pressure ulcers)
(D) Dimethicone Protectant applied
(E) Zinc oxide applied
(F) Physician notified
(G) Tegaderm or Flexigel applied
(H) Other

Staging Pressure Ulcers

Stage 1 Persistent non blanchable erythema of intact skin. Individuals with darker skin may present with red, blue or purplish discoloration of the skin. Warmth, edema, induration or hardness may also be indicators.

Stage 2 Partial thickness skin loss involving the epidermis, dermis or both. Present as a superficial abrasion, blister or shallow crater.

Stage 3 Full thickness skin loss involving damage necrosis of the subcutaneous tissue. May extend down to, but not through, the underlying fascia.

Stage 4 Full thickness skin loss with extensive destruction, tissue necrosis or damage to underlying muscle, bone or supporting structures.

Nonstageable Wound covered with nonvariable tissue such as eschar. Deep purple discoloration of wounds may indicate deeper tissue damage

Initials	Signature/Title	Print Name	Initials	Signature/Title	Print Name

for skin impairment. The next three phases of the PDCA model—Do, Check, Act—demonstrate the particulars of the improvements gained in prevention of HAPUs and are detailed on pages 88 and 89.

Conclusions and Implications

Throughout this journey, CCHS has embraced the idea that a zero tolerance for hospital-acquired pressure ulcers is achievable, which is a significant culture change for every direct care nurse in the system. Evidence supports that this goal can only be sustained through the daily vigilance of skin surveillance. Without frequent and routine surveillance and assessment, a firm belief that "what we do" can make a difference, and the involvement of the entire team, all other preventive efforts can be meaningless. Hospital-wide multidisciplinary teams and unit-based teams are absolutely necessary to accomplish and sustain success in the prevention of skin breakdown. In MICU, patients do have many contributing factors that make them at high risk for breakdown, but MICU staff alone cannot achieve success in reducing and preventing skin breakdown. It takes an entire healthcare system to work cohesively as a team across every single nursing unit to provide the optimal outcomes that patients expect at Christiana Care Health System. No patient deserves a hospital-acquired infection.

Sharing NDNQI Data with Bedside Nurses Leads to Improved Skin Integrity

Janet Doyle-Munoz, RN, BSN, CWOCN
Wound and Ostomy Nurse
Janet.Munoz@atlantichealth.org

Toni McTigue, APRN, BC,CWOCN
Wound, Ostomy, and Continence Nurse

Cynthia Abline, RN
Manager, Quality and Outcomes Management

Bonnie Forshner, RN, BSN, CCRN
Unit Educator

Morristown Memorial Hospital—Morristown, New Jersey

Editors' pick:

INSIGHTS & IDEAS FROM THIS FACILITY

Moved to unit-specific data with NDNQI and instituted practice changes on a problem unit which led to improvements.

Facility Summary

Facility	Morristown Memorial Hospital—Morristown, New Jersey **www.morristownmemorialhospital.org**
Facility setting	Morristown Memorial Hospital (MMH) is a nonprofit, community-based acute care teaching hospital located in suburban northwest New Jersey.
Teaching status	Teaching hospital
Ownership status	Nonprofit
Community demographics	• Morris County is the county seat; 25 miles west of New York City. • Population (2000) 410,212. • Third among the highest median income U.S. counties, 10th by per capita income; approx. 3.0% of the population below the poverty line. • 87.20% Caucasian, 2.80 % African American; Asian, 0.04%; approx. 8% Hispanic; 0.12% Native American; 6.26% Pacific Islander.
Number of hospital staffed beds	564 inpatient beds
Indicators used	Nursing Care Hours; Patient Days; Patient falls; Pressure Ulcers; RN Education
System or unit improved	Cardiac care unit and neuro–special care unit
Indicator(s) improved	Hospital acquired pressure ulcer
QI report card/ document used	NDNQI quarterly reports and hospital-developed, nurse–sensitive report card
NDNQI participant since	2004
Magnet™ status	Redesignation 2005

UNIT PROFILE: CCU

Unit sizes and types	• Cardiac care unit: 8 beds • Neuro-special care unit: 5 beds
Unit RN staff profile	• RN staff provides approx. 95% of total nursing hours • 58% of RN staff have BSN or greater. • 28% of RN staff has current national certification in specialty area.
Skill mix of RNs, other personnel	• 5–6% of patient care provided by unlicensed assistive personnel.
Organizational structure of unit	Nursing manager ⟶ Clinical coordinator ⟶ Unit educator ⟶ Staff nurse ⟶ Nursing assistant

UNIT PROFILE: NEURO-SPECIAL UNIT

Unit size and type	Five-bed neuro-special care unit
Unit RN staff profile	• RN staff provides nearly 94% of total nursing hours • 78% of RN staff has BSN or greater • 11% of RN staff has current national certification in specialty area
Skill mix of RNs, other personnel	• 6–7% of patient care supplied by unlicensed assistive personnel
Organizational structure of unit	Nursing manager ⟶ Clinical coordinator ⟶ Unit educator ⟶ Staff nurse ⟶ Nursing assistant

Sharing NDNQI Data with Bedside Nurses Leads to Improved Skin Integrity

Janet Doyle-Munoz, RN, BSN, CWOCN
Wound and Ostomy Nurse
Janet.Munoz@atlantichealth.org

Toni McTigue, APRN, BC,CWOCN
Wound, Ostomy, and Continence Nurse

Cynthia Abline, RN
Manager, Quality and Outcomes Management

Bonnie Forshner, RN, BSN, CCRN
Unit Educator

Introductory Summary

Morristown Memorial Hospital (MMH) is a non-profit, community-based 564-bed acute care teaching hospital located in suburban northwest New Jersey. The American Nurses Credentialing Commission awarded MMH Magnet designation in 2001 and 2005. MMH has been serving the community for more than 100 years, setting high standards for patient care in state-of-the-art facilities with a full range of medical specialties and services. It is a Level 1 Regional Trauma Center designated by the American College of Surgeons and has the largest cardiac surgery center in the state as well as a Level III Regional Perinatal Center.

MMH is staffed with two wound, ostomy, and continence clinicians. These clinicians play a vital role in establishing, monitoring, and evaluating wound care standards and patient care guidelines. Evidence-based practice provides the foundation for sound clinical decisions, patient advocacy, and nursing education. Select professional nurses from each nursing unit are given special education in the management of patients with wounds and are designated as the unit wound care coordinator. They serve as champions and resources for peers on their individual units.

The hospital has a proud history of empowering its nursing staff to participate in decision-making in regards to their practice using the shared governance model. Shared governance allows for the communication of data along the organizational structure to help facilitate change at the unit level. Communication starts at the top with the CEO of Atlantic Health system, of which MMH is a part, and travels down to the chief nursing officer. The CNO is also a voting member of the medical staff, which gives nursing a voice in decision-making in the upper levels of the organization.

NDNQI Startup Considerations

The opportunity to participate in the NDNQI offered MMH the ability to compare itself to national benchmarks at the unit level. It acknowledged that as an acute care facility, the hospital exceeds minimum standards and demonstrates excellence in nursing. MMH has been conducting organizational pressure ulcer prevalence studies since 1996 on an annual basis. While this provided a global annual prevalence rate, it did not provide unit-specific data. Advantages of NDNQI participation included quarterly prevalence studies and unit-specific benchmarks. No additional resources were required but the wound care coordinators received special training to collect the data. This education included an intensive five-module program and exam. Teaching included the use of the Braden scale, pressure ulcer prevention, pressure ulcer staging, and treatment and documentation. Wound care rounds, with hands-on education, were given on individual units to reinforce classroom learning.

Quality Measurement and Reporting

Data are collected on a quarterly basis and submitted to NDNQI. Data indicators include:

- Current Braden scale score
- Prior risk assessment score

- Recency of prior risk assessment (hours)
- Patient at risk status
- Documentation of prevention protocol
- Pressure ulcer stages
- Identification of the pressure ulcer as facility acquired or present on admission

NDNQI then generates a report for the organization that compares MMH to national benchmarks. This report is categorized according to the unit's specialty, such as adult critical care, adult step-down, adult medical, adult surgical, and adult combined med–surg in the 500+-bed category. The NDNQI data are disseminated to the Shared Governance Quality Improvement Council, unit nursing managers, unit-based quality improvement councils, and the pressure ulcer subcommittee which is composed of the unit wound care coordinators.

Action plans are developed in collaboration with wound specialists tailored for individual units using Plan-Do-Study-Act (PDSA) improvement methodology. In addition, changes to evidence-based best practices are brought to Shared Governance Practice Council for approval.

Quality Improvement: Results from Data Collection

Trending results tabulated from the raw NDNQI data for 2004 and compared to 2005, revealed the following (Figure 1):

- Overall hospital-wide percentage of patients with hospital-acquired pressure ulcers (all stages) dropped from 10.9% in 2004 to 9.5% in 2005
- Percentage of patients with a Stage II or greater hospital-acquired pressure ulcers dropped from 6.2% in 2004 to 4.1% in 2005

Transforming Nursing Data Into Quality Care:
Profiles of Quality Improvement in U.S. Healthcare Facilities

Collection of NDNQI data has allowed the wound care clinicians to target nursing units with patients who were at high risk for pressure ulcer development. Wound care clinicians, in collaboration with the pressure ulcer subcommittee, developed a global interventional action plan. The committee used evidence-based practice standards for the prevention and treatment of pressure ulcers based on the recommendations of the National Pressure Ulcer Advisory Panel (NPUAP), the Wound, Ostomy, and Continence Society, and the U.S. Agency for Healthcare Research and Quality (AHRQ).

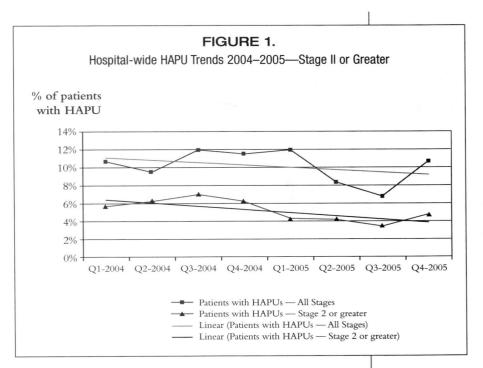

FIGURE 1.
Hospital-wide HAPU Trends 2004–2005—Stage II or Greater

Quality Improvement: Hospital-wide

Hospital-wide interventions included:

- Revision of wound care protocol to evidence-based practice guidelines,

- Intensive education of unit-based wound care coordinators, emphasizing the use of the Braden scale, prevention measures, pressure ulcer staging, and treatment,

- Development of wound care clinician triggers for Stage I pressure ulcers or greater,

- Changing the Braden scale assessment from weekly to daily and changing definition of patient at risk from a Braden score of 14 to a Braden score of 18 or below,

- Development of system-wide wound and ostomy intranet web site, and

- Development of Braden scale and wound care competencies for professional and nonprofessional staff.

Preliminary results of 2004 NDNQI data analyses demonstrated pressure ulcer rates that were above the national mean in isolated nursing units at MMH. However, as a result of the efforts described above, along with unit-specific interventions, several nursing units have achieved outstanding outcomes in 2005.

Quality Improvement: Cardiac Care

The cardiac care unit (CCU) is an eight-bed teaching unit that meets the health care needs of critically ill medical cardiac patients. Patient diagnoses cover a diverse cross-section of acute cardiac issues, including myocardial infarction, congestive heart failure, cardiogenic shock, ventilator-dependent respiratory failure, and post-cardiac arrest. As a result of the complexity of care that these patients require, they are often relatively immobile and on bed rest for several days or even weeks. Accordingly, the staff in the CCU must be vigilant at preserving skin integrity and promoting pressure ulcer prevention. The staff have initiated the following measures to accomplish those goals:

- Multiple signs permanently posted in the charting area of the nursing station serve as a constant

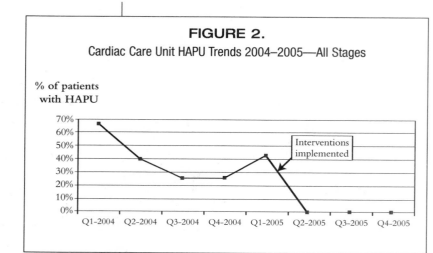

FIGURE 2.

Cardiac Care Unit HAPU Trends 2004–2005—All Stages

% of patients with HAPU

Interventions implemented

reminder to staff to call in a wound care consult if a patient has a Stage I or greater pressure ulcer, new ostomy, existing ostomy with difficulties, or specialty bed questions.

- Braden skin risk assessment done daily on all patients. For any patient identified with a Braden score of 18 or below, a pressure ulcer prevention protocol is instituted along with notification to the wound care department.

- In addition to the wound and ostomy nurse, the CCU staff directly utilizes the unit-based wound care coordinator for informal consults and recommendations for pressure ulcer prevention and treatment at the bedside.

- The CCU purchased six wedge pillows to facilitate repositioning of patients at least every two hours.

- Heel lift suspension boots are applied to all patients who require long-term immobilization, present with a high Braden score (10–12), or already have a Stage I pressure ulcer or greater.

- Purchase of pressure redistribution support beds with lateral rotation for all CCU beds.

- All urinary and fecal incontinence are treated with periwash spray and a barrier protectant cream. Open Absorb-Plus mattress pads are used to contain incontinence instead of diapers.• Any patient who

has two or more episodes of diarrhea in a 24-hour period gets a fecal incontinence collection system.

- Weekly pre-albumin levels and nutritional consults done on all patients who have pressure ulcers, are immobile, or are on mechanical ventilation.

- Head of bed is limited to 30° or less to prevent skin shearing.

- Staff are continually updated and educated on the latest wound care trends and treatments via educational bulletin board with postings during annual training competencies.

As a result in the first quarter of 2005, the CCU had a hospital-acquired pressure ulcer prevalence rate of 43%. For the remainder of 2005, the unit had a hospital-acquired rate of 0% (Figure 2).

Quality Improvement: Neuro-special Care

Neuro-special care (NSC) is a five-bed unit composed of patients who have critical neurological diagnoses that include trauma, medical, autoimmune, and post-surgical neurological disorders. Patients are immobile for long periods of time due to paralysis, respiratory insufficiency, and altered or loss of consciousness. Skin care is a top priority with the staff. Prevention interventions include:

- Skin assessment and inspection are done every shift and documented in the nursing record.

- Nutritional consult done within 24 hours of admission to unit.

- Weekly pre-albumin levels to assess and monitor nutritional status.

- Pressure redistribution support surfaces for all NSC beds.

- Strict monitoring of patients hydration status by hourly intake and outputs and basic metabolic panel monitoring.

- Meticulous turning and positioning every two hours.
- Education of staff by unit wound care coordinator on regular basis about risk assessment, prevention. and treatment of pressure ulcers.
- Patient is moved out of bed as soon as possible to chair.

The prevalence rate for hospital-acquired pressure ulcers in the NSC was 20% in the first quarter of 2005 and 0% for the remainder of 2005 (Figure 3). Dramatic fluctuations in the run chart are attributed to the small unit size for NSC. Because this is a five-bed unit, one patient with a pressure ulcer can affect the data significantly.

Common themes shared by both CCU and NSC units include low patient–nurse ratios, consistent skin assessment, and pressure ulcer prevention and wound care practices. Most importantly, the unit wound care coordinators were instrumental in serving as role models and mentors for their peers.

Lessons Learned

Pressure ulcer prevention is a patient safety goal at Morristown Memorial Hospital. Integrating the NDNQI data collection system to predict pressure ulcer prevalence affords MMH the ability to monitor pressure ulcer development on a consistent basis. The bedside nurse becomes an integral part of the data collection process, which provides feedback to nurses at the bedside. It is an important part of planning and implementing an effective pressure ulcer program. According to one NSC nurse, "Skin care is a priority that is as important as monitoring a patient's vital signs."

Limitations of data collection include patients being transferred into the unit with a pre-existing pressure ulcer, dietary constraints, and a computerized charting

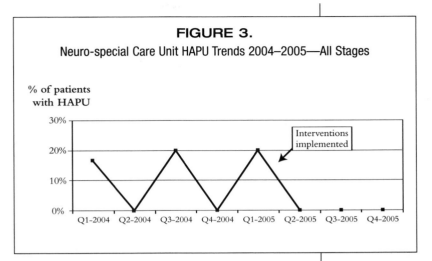

FIGURE 3.

Neuro-special Care Unit HAPU Trends 2004–2005—All Stages

% of patients with HAPU

system. Data collection was performed by an RN who was specialty trained in data collection methods, pressure ulcer identification, and staging. The nurse was also a member of the unit in which the study was conducted. We are in the process of working with senior management to change the method of data collection thus decreasing bias and limiting variables.

Conclusions and Implications

In response to the increase in HAPU trends during fourth quarter 2005, the pressure ulcer program was re-evaluated and a multidisciplinary committee was established. Action plans will be developed based on the recommendations from the committee and data from the NDNQI quarterly surveys. NDNQI data have allowed the committee to monitor individual unit progress and focus limited resources in the appropriate and most effective manner.

In conclusion, the NDNQI methodology has facilitated the introduction of pressure ulcers as a quality indicator at MMH. This structure provides MMH the opportunity to highlight the implementation of pressure ulcer prevention strategies. It empowers the bedside nurse to provide superior nursing care, set goals, and test changes in clinical practice.

Quality Report Cards Inform Staff Nurses About Pressure Ulcer Rates and Document Success of Quality Improvement Initiatives

Margaret Talley, RN, CNS, CWCN
District Wound Clinical Nurse Specialist
margaret.talley@pph.org

Ann Moore, RN, MN, CWCN
Program Director, Wound and Hyperbaric Clinic

Eva Krall, RN, MN, CNS
Pomerado Medical Surgical CNS

Palomar Pomerado Health Hospital District—Poway and Escondido, California

Editors' pick:

INSIGHTS & IDEAS FROM THIS FACILITY

"Cheerleading" and RNs educating aides on their role in good outcomes led to improvements. QI initiatives must be kept in the foreground for ongoing success.

Facility Summary

Facility	Palomar Pomerado Health Hospital District— Poway and Escondido, California http://www.pph.org
Facility setting	Rural north San Diego; average household income $47,000.
Teaching status	Non-teaching hospital
Ownership status	Community owned
Community demographics	Retirees, mixed cultural group, Hispanic 50%, and high growth rate 9%
Number of hospital staffed beds	• Palomar 319 • Pomerado 107
Unit size and type	• Palomar: CCU–35, IMC–32, Tele–30, T-8-33, T-7-33, T-5-32 • Pomerado: ICU–12, IMC–8, MST–34, MS–18
Indicators used	Hospital acquired pressure ulcers
System or unit improved	System-wide across these units
Indicator(s) improved	Hospital acquired pressure ulcers Stage II plus
QI report card/ document used	Focus PDCA
NDNQI participant since	2003
Magnet™ status	Application sent 2005

UNIT PROFILE

Unit size and type	See above
Unit RN staff profile	CCU and ICU—2:1; Tele and IMC—3:1 or 4:1; Med–Surg—5:1 with nursing assistants
Unit skill mix of RNs, other personnel	Nursing assistants used mostly on med–surg units only. Assistants used for lifting and bathing on other units.
Organizational structure of unit	Staff, charge nurses, shift supervisors (2), managers or directors

Transforming Nursing Data Into Quality Care:
Profiles of Quality Improvement in U.S. Healthcare Facilities

Quality Report Cards Inform Staff Nurses About Pressure Ulcer Rates and Document Success of Quality Improvement Initiatives

Margaret Talley, RN, CNS, CWCN
District Wound Clinical Nurse Specialist
margaret.talley@pph.org

Ann Moore, RN, MN, CWCN
Program Director, Wound and Hyperbaric Clinic

Eva Krall, RN, MN, CNS
Pomerado Medical Surgical CNS

Introductory Summary

The Palomar Pomerado Health (PPH) hospital district in the North San Diego area is the largest public district hospital in California.

The initiation of the collection of prevalence data began in 2001. The manager of the outpatient wound clinic noticed a number of patients being admitted to the outpatient wound care clinic that were previous health system patients. She suspected the health system had a high prevalence of pressure ulcers and initiated a prevalence study process. At that time, studies were executed with the assistance of a national bed company.

Results of these studies validated a higher than the national average rate for hospital-acquired pressure ulcers. The hospital then hired a clinical nurse specialist certified in wound care to assist in the improvement of patient care to reduce the prevalence of hospital-acquired pressure ulcers.

Concurrently, the health system was moving toward participation in the Magnet designation process. The Nursing Database for Nursing Quality Indicators (NDNQI) was selected to collect unit-based, nurse-sensitive quality indicators. At least one year's worth of data is needed before Magnet application. The Palomar Pomerado Health System has been participating in NDNQI Pressure Ulcer data collection since 2003 and submitted a Magnet application in 2006.

One of the indicators in NDNQI is the prevalence of hospital-acquired pressure ulcers. The hospital already had these data as well as a functional team to continue with the quality improvement process and opportunity.

Pressure Ulcer Prevalence:

Facility at a Glance

The Palomar Pomerado Health hospital district covers the 800-square mile, semi-rural, and suburban North Inland San Diego area and is the largest public district hospital in California. The community is close to the Mexican border and interregional commuting from Baja California results in culturally diverse patient population. Additionally, there are many retirement communities nearby.

It is a non-teaching, nonprofit health system. In addition to the two acute care hospitals, the system includes a wound clinic, outpatient surgicenter, home health agency, and two skilled nursing facilities.

Active team members in the pressure ulcer prevalence reduction project are RNs from all the hospitals as well as the home health agency. The pressure ulcer prevalence improvement occurred within both acute care hospitals. Active RN team members are from the following units:

Palomar Medical Center (319 staffed beds):

- 35-bed mixed Critical Care Unit with 1:1 or 1:2 RN-to-patient ratio

- 32-monitored-bed Intermediate Care unit with 1:3 ratio

- Progressive Cardiac Telemetry Unit with a 1:4 ratio

- 33-bed Medical Oncology unit (T-7) with a 1:5 ratio

- 33-bed Surgical Unit (T-8) with a ratio of one RN or LVN to 5 patients

- 32-bed Ortho Unit(T-5) has telemetry capacity with a 1:5 ratio

Pomerado Hospital (107 staffed beds):

- 12-bed Intensive Care Unit with a 1:2 RN-to-patient ratio

- 8-bed IMC Geriatric and Bariatric Unit staffed with a 1:4 ratio

- 34-bed Medical-Surgical Telemetry and 18-bed surgical and medical overflow units with a 1:5 ratio in both units

NDNQI Startup Considerations

When Palomar Pomerado Health (PPH) began collecting and reporting NDNQI Hospital-Acquired Pressure Ulcer (HAPU) data in 2003, it became apparent that the district's two hospitals had a much higher pressure ulcer prevalence rate than the national comparison.

The HAPU indicator was targeted for improvement, particularly for our at-risk population. Initially, data collection was done by the wound clinic wound-certified RNs with minimal staff involvement on any of the units. In a 1:1 mentoring process with the unit team members, the RN team members from each unit became responsible for data collection and prevalence assessment with a clinic wound-certified RN. By June 2005, skin team members were competent to independently perform pressure ulcer prevalence assessment and data collection. A minimum of two wound-certified nurses were available to validate pressure ulcer findings or suspicions for team members during the study at each site.

One of the first activities the team engaged in was a skin and incontinence product trial (Talley and Moore 2006). The team chose the new product and a large-scale education program was rolled out to the units. There were many opportunities for staff to review educational materials aimed at correctly identifying and treating incontinence-related skin problems.

For the next project, the team identified inadequate documentation on community acquired pressure ulcers, which was reflected in unit prevalence rates. Accurate identification and documentation of these ulcers would yield an immediate reduction in ulcer rates and prompt ulcer care. The team also identified a need for all bedside staff to be able to accurately assess skin and stage lesions. This became one of the second major educational endeavors for the skin team. The computerized charting system was modified to fully capture pressure ulcers during admission assessment. During prevalence study data collection, adherence to complete and accurate skin assessment was audited and discrepancies investigated and resolved, if possible.

Strategies to Gain Buy-In and Engage Staff in Process

Skin became a major initiative for the nursing division in spring 2005. The major strategy adopted to assure success in pressure ulcer prevention is to gain and sustain engagement of bedside caregivers in the process. Methods included development of the skin team, with membership from each of the nursing units. The team meets monthly at both facilities and meetings are teleconferenced to support attendance and communication. Skin team members then report NDNQI data to both unit and system-wide professional practice councils. Skin care remains in the forefront with placement on our quality indicator scorecard. With the daily assessment, skin is emphasized with the "ABCS" (Airway, Breathing, Circulation, SKIN) of patient assessment.

New staff are introduced to skin care upon hire, with skin care basics and NDNQI data presented in the nursing orientation. On participating units, staff are provided with quarterly updates of both formal and informal education classes. Wound care specialists (wound care CNS and wound clinic physician) support staff-run patient case studies. Case presentations start with staff members presenting their patient in an informal forum on the unit and ends with the team rounding at the bedside so the patient can participate in the plan of care.

Quality Measurement and Reporting

Palomar Pomerado utilizes a Balanced Scorecard method in order to focus on key strategic objectives that are considered important to the system's future success. The nursing division leadership decided to focus on nurse-sensitive NDNQI measures of quality, which included distressingly high HAPU rates. The strategic goal was to reduce these rates and report improvement activities back to leadership. At PPH, the nursing leadership division's objective for the Balanced Scorecard report for the period 2005–2006 was to reduce HAPU rates. Managers, clinical leaders, and skin team members were charged with creating incentives, support, and initiatives to facilitate successful strategies to address this issue. The features of this scorecard and its function in the PPH "roadmap to success" are shown in Figure 1.

The Nursing Quality Education and Research Department at Palomar Pomerado exists to address nursing quality issues and facilitate American Nurse Credentialing Center (ANCC) Magnet designation. To assist each unit and each skin team member with a consistent mechanism for organization of their pressure ulcer reduction efforts, a quality measurement report card was developed by the Nursing Quality Education and Research Department. This report card was used to communicate to participating units our initiatives and progress. Immediately following each prevalence study, the unit CNS, wound care CNS, and skin team members evaluate findings, develop a plan for improvement, and communicate with staff members.

Quality Improvement of HAPU Indicator

Palomar Pomerado Health (PPH) utilized the Plan Do Check Act (PDCA) framework for quality improvement, which led to positive outcomes in the reduction of hospital-acquired pressure ulcers within the entire PPH healthcare system.

Pressure Ulcer Prevalence:

Quality Report Cards Inform Staff Nurses About Pressure Ulcer Rates and Document Success of Quality Improvement Initiatives

109

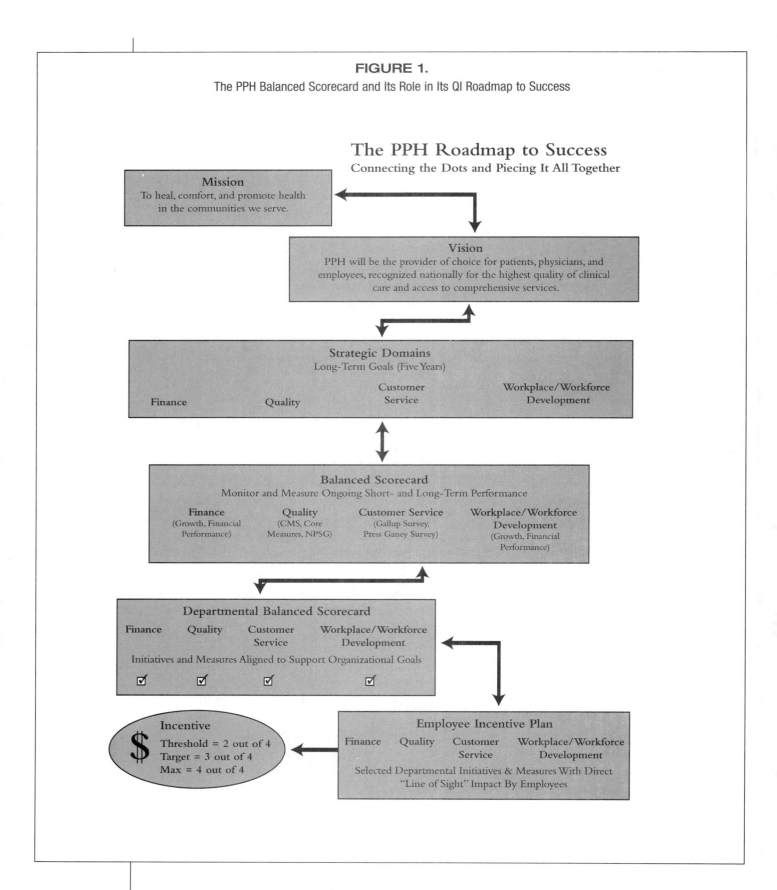

FIGURE 1.

The PPH Balanced Scorecard and Its Role in Its QI Roadmap to Success

The PPH Roadmap to Success
Connecting the Dots and Piecing It All Together

Mission
To heal, comfort, and promote health in the communities we serve.

Vision
PPH will be the provider of choice for patients, physicians, and employees, recognized nationally for the highest quality of clinical care and access to comprehensive services.

Strategic Domains
Long–Term Goals (Five Years)

Finance   Quality   Customer Service   Workplace/Workforce Development

Balanced Scorecard
Monitor and Measure Ongoing Short- and Long-Term Performance

Finance (Growth, Financial Performance)   Quality (CMS, Core Measures, NPSG)   Customer Service (Gallup Survey, Press Ganey Survey)   Workplace/Workforce Development (Growth, Financial Performance)

Departmental Balanced Scorecard
Finance   Quality   Customer Service   Workplace/Workforce Development

Initiatives and Measures Aligned to Support Organizational Goals

☑   ☑   ☑   ☑

Incentive
$ Threshold = 2 out of 4
Target = 3 out of 4
Max = 4 out of 4

Employee Incentive Plan
Finance   Quality   Customer Service   Workplace/Workforce Development

Selected Departmental Initiatives & Measures With Direct "Line of Sight" Impact By Employees

The graphs of these outcomes over time (Figures 2, 3, and 4) show the latest NDNQI executive summary comparing both Palomar Hospital's critical care, step-down, and medical surgical units and Pomerado Hospitals critical care and medical unit HAPU trends. Staff utilize the findings as baseline data before implementing skin team change projects and to evaluate the project outcomes post-implementation. The trends can also point to problem areas that require creative solutions by skin team staff as HAPU trends start to creep up (as shown in the second graph in Figure 3 on Palomar Hospital's stepdown trends).

The facilitation and support of an engaged skin team, with representatives from each clinical unit, were integral to the success of the process. The team participated in revision and implementation of a new evidence-based integumentary nursing standard of care.

Additionally, the team co-developed, with the wound care center, standardized order sets for pressure ulcer care and system standardization of the wound care product formulary, resulting in system continuity of care. Changes in use of skin product prevention, in servicing and the removal of plastic-coated drawsheets and replacing them with a strong absorbent under-pad/lift sheet named the "GeriChux," yielded continued reductions in hospital-acquired pressure ulcers. (Figure 5 shows the PDCA cycle report from one unit's pilot trial study of such a product replacement, which was eventually adopted system-wide.) PDCA was the template for the quality change while the system change theory of William Bridges (1990) describes staff engagement in the integration of the desired practice behavior into patient care.

In addition, another element that continues to strengthen the outcomes for the process is the collaborative relationship with the outpatient wound care clinic. Collaboration is demonstrated in the establishment of inpatient wound care rounds performed by the medical director of the Center for Wound Care and Hyperbaric Medicine. Staff identify wound patients and the wound care physician, in collaboration with

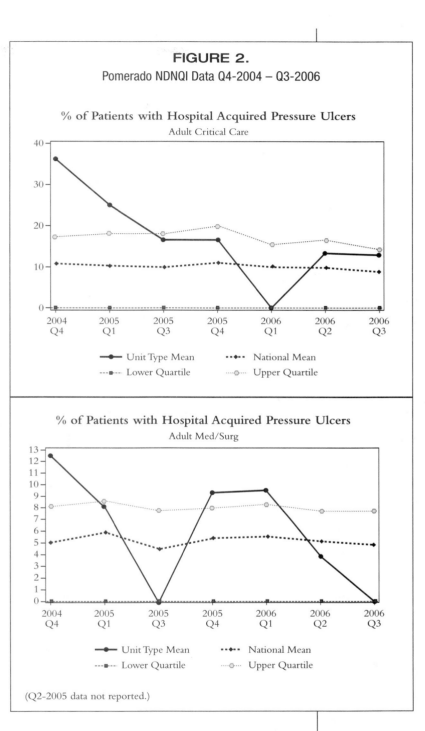

FIGURE 2.

Pomerado NDNQI Data Q4-2004 – Q3-2006

% of Patients with Hospital Acquired Pressure Ulcers
Adult Critical Care

% of Patients with Hospital Acquired Pressure Ulcers
Adult Med/Surg

(Q2-2005 data not reported.)

the wound CNS, performs a consult. The physician and CNS then discuss the plan of care with rationale to the staff and turn the consult into a teaching opportunity for all caregivers. This interaction provides a link between the inpatient and outpatient care of patients with wounds.

Pressure Ulcer Prevalence:

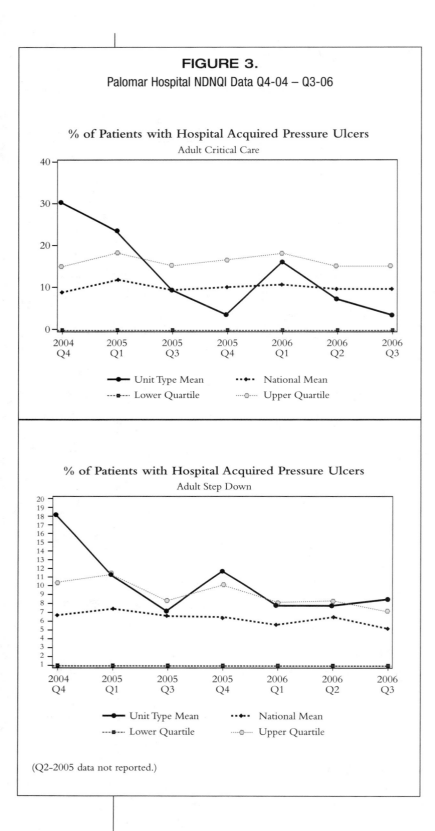

FIGURE 3.
Palomar Hospital NDNQI Data Q4-04 – Q3-06

% of Patients with Hospital Acquired Pressure Ulcers
Adult Critical Care

| | 2004 Q4 | 2005 Q1 | 2005 Q3 | 2005 Q4 | 2006 Q1 | 2006 Q2 | 2006 Q3 |

Legend:
— Unit Type Mean
···•··· National Mean
---■--- Lower Quartile
····○···· Upper Quartile

% of Patients with Hospital Acquired Pressure Ulcers
Adult Step Down

Legend:
— Unit Type Mean
---■--- Lower Quartile
···•··· National Mean
····○···· Upper Quartile

(Q2-2005 data not reported.)

Quality Improvement of HAPU Indicator: How the Facility Uses the Data and How the Facility Reacted

The PPH skin team at both facilities continue to use NDNQI data to evaluate the individual and group projects designed to reduce pressure ulcer prevalence. The individual unit and associated skin team members pilot various evidence-based projects and when successful, mentor other units with successful change projects. An example of one of these change projects conducted in a critical care unit is illustrated in the PDCA process improvement format that was published in the PPH nursing newsletter and presented as a poster at the San Diego Association of California Nurse Leaders (ACNL) conference August 2006 (Figure 5). These projects provide the hospital system with evidence of Magnet-caliber nursing and the opportunity to showcase nursing commitment to the hospital community through reporting to the district board. Skin team nurse members also have opportunities to showcase their unit projects with poster submissions at professional organization meetings.

Units utilize strategies specific to their practice areas. Something that works for one unit may or may not be useful in a different practice setting depending on patient population or staffing mix. Examples of strategies used on the medical surgical units include leading weekly manager/CNS skin rounds, interventions directed by Braden reports, or biweekly pressure ulcer assessment, measurement, and treatments provided by skin team members. In the medical surgical unit, staff are provided with a feedback sheet if they cannot be present when rounds are conducted. This enhances communication so the entire team is aware of patient findings and interventions. On all units, staff participation is supported in conducting prevalence studies, with ancillary staff involvement to assist with the process as well as to provide educational support to others who are in contact with the patient.

Committed skin team staff are recognized for their involvement by presentations with embroidered lab coats. Units with sustained improvement in NDNQI prevalence rates over two quarters are given pizza parties. Rewards are an important part of celebrating the team's success.

Lessons Learned

The team developed a greater appreciation for the change process within a large healthcare district as well as garnered respect for each other's strengths. The recognition of the need to have a well-defined plan at the initiation of the project is important to assure success, along with the flexibility to change the plan as needed. To sustain motivation and enthusiasm, "cheerleading" was encouraged and utilized.

Among the more pleasant surprises during this period was the individual growth seen in even the quietest of skin team members through their presentations to leadership. Staff created a network sharing information amongst themselves and units. The endless enthusiasm shown by the ICU skin team and their tenacity at sticking to the pilot program that often felt "like it went on forever," was truly remarkable as was the team's ability to act as champions for system change by sharing their knowledge with other units across the system. Administrative support, enthusiasm, and the rewards for sustained positive outcomes, as well as staff willingness to take on challenging projects, provided us with ongoing motivation.

Also unforeseen, but more problematic, was what occurred during the initial training pertaining to skin care product use and targeting the wrong group. RNs did not go back and educate their nurse aide partners as anticipated. CNA change champions needed identification and training, so the process would extend to all bedside caregivers. Nurse aides are often the first to identify skin issues and intervene. Enhanced RN-to-nurse aide communication was facilitated by skin team members modeling the desired behavior during rounds.

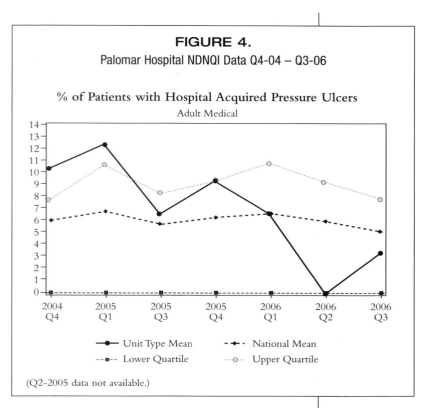

FIGURE 4.
Palomar Hospital NDNQI Data Q4-04 – Q3-06

% of Patients with Hospital Acquired Pressure Ulcers
Adult Medical

— Unit Type Mean   — National Mean
— Lower Quartile   — Upper Quartile

(Q2-2005 data not available.)

Other challenges included delays where units took longer to implement the new skin care products. These unit team members did not have the educational skills, lacked supervisor support, or had trouble communicating needs to a dedicated central supply supervisor. Census fluctuation also created problems when staff were spread too thin to attend training or were rotated to other units and missed educational sessions. Some RN skin assessment skills were not strong and initial tissue injury was missed or inaccurately staged. Ongoing inter-rater reliability testing, with a poster session prior to each study, has improved new skin team members' pressure ulcer assessment skills.

Among the more predictable variables in such a process of change were such barriers to change as indifferent ancillary participants, differences in unit enthusiasm, and lack of support in such ancillary areas as central supply. Sometimes broken or inefficient equipment and supplies (i.e., support surfaces) contributed to loss of an opportunity to initiate optimal pressure ulcer prevention. Staff movement/transfer and loss of skin team

Pressure Ulcer Prevalence:

Quality Report Cards Inform Staff Nurses About Pressure Ulcer Rates and Document Success of Quality Improvement Initiatives   **113**

members should be expected as well. All of these problems and their resolution continue to be addressed within the context of the skin team.

Currently, the skin initiative must always be present in the foreground and incorporated as a quality measure and incentive plan. Maintaining and sustaining interest and enthusiasm is an ongoing challenge.

Among the predictable costs for start-up were paying staff to participate in quarterly prevalence studies as well as attendance at monthly two-hour skin team meetings, all of which were budgeted into labor costs and unproductive time. When census is low, staffing is usually adjusted to the change in volume. This practice was tested when the skin team meetings were maintained during a lean census period, and leadership stayed committed to support the meetings.

Other costs were driven by each unit, and the model that the unit put into place to address the skin initiative was ongoing. Units varied in budgeting 2 to 12 hours weekly for skin followup on their individual units. To save costs, units with multiple skin team members only sent one representative to the monthly meeting, who reported back to their peers.

There were also potential savings in streamlining the wound and skin product formulary as well as monitoring and standardizing support surface use. The skin team implemented the streamlined formulary and developed a new support surface decision tree to guide bed utilization. As well, there was an overall reduction in linen cost for the hospital when the thick and heavy "geripads" were eliminated.

It is imperative to be able to utilize NDNQI nurse-sensitive indicators to keep prevention successes visible to hospital administrators. Bedside staff are best suited to evaluate and improve bedside care when supported and mentored by advanced practice nursing and leadership.

Conclusions and Implications

Development and support of a strong, nurse-led team dedicated to improving bedside skin care can yield impressive sustained reductions in hospital-acquired pressure ulcers within a large healthcare system. A strong commitment by staff and leadership is essential but there is also an element of creativity that needs to be fostered and nurtured by nurse mentors and experts in pressure ulcer prevention and care. NDNQI data are shared throughout the organization and staff takes a keen interest in the latest pressure ulcer rates for their units. When there is a rise in hospital-acquired pressure ulcers within the unit, staff will redouble their efforts to find ways to address the problem.

In this environment, skin team experts have to be easily available to staff for bedside assessment and planning. The staff need to have the ability to evaluate new products, support surfaces, and supplies within the context of their unit and work environment. They also need to have access to the wound care and clinical nurse specialists who are able to advise them on steps to market changes within the healthcare system to improve practice. Once the cycle of improvement has been implemented, it is much easier to sustain. New skin team members rotate into the group and are mentored by seasoned members. Members leave to pursue new opportunities on other units yet they retain their skill and expertise in skin assessment. The entire organization benefited from this teamwork experience.

References

Bridges, W. Managing transitions in complex change efforts. *Surviving Corporate Transition*. New York: Doubleday Books; 1988.

Talley, M.E., & Moore A.Z.. An integrated health system endeavor to reduce the prevalence of hospital-acquired pressure ulcers. Abstract and Poster Presentation 1709. 38th Annual Wound Ostomy and Continence Nurses Society Annual Conference, Minneapolis: June 2006.

FIGURE 5.

PDCA Case Study—Palomar Hospital Critical Care Unit

Palomar Hospital CCU Change Project (Adapted System-wide)— Quality Improvement in Action: Geripad vs. Chux

Margaret Talley, RN, CNS, CWCN; Linda S. Olson, RN; and Debbie Nelson, RN, BSN

August 11, 2006

Find: There is an opportunity to optimize the therapeutic properties of existing support surfaces and reduce linen use at the Palomar Pomerado Health (PPH) hospital district.

Organize: Two groups, PPH skin team and advanced practice nurse teams, exist and are functional with active representation. There is synergy toward a common evidence-based practice goal.

Clarify: PPH owns beds with pressure and friction reduction surfaces. Current practice reveals that staff layer the beds with thick geripad linen, mitigating the pressure and friction reduction capabilities of the surfaces. Pressure ulcer prevalence rates are higher than national benchmarks on units where this occurs. Concurrently, linen costs are rising.

Understand: Units have different staff levels; some have all RNs others have RN/hospital assistant mixes. Stakeholders include managers, EVS, SPD, RNs and hospital assistants.

Select: A literature search was done supporting the removal of layers between the patient and the therapeutic support surface and presented to the skin team and advanced practice nurse group. The skin team and advance practice nurses agree that geripad removal would benefit patient skin. Alternative absorbent chux would be needed for incontinent patients.

Plan: Two CCU skin team members championed a pilot in the 36-bed CCU. The project met needs of both skin team RNs who were actively seeking BSN and MSN advancement and academic projects. Additionally, skin team members from all units were anxious to find Performance Enhancement Program (PEP) activities that would provide a financial bonus. Geripad teaching projects were completed by team members and shared with staff on their units.

Do: Implementation ideas and barriers were shared with the wound CNS and skin team members at monthly meetings. Several chux products were tried and evaluated by CCU staff for durability and absorbency. CCU staff also tried alternate draw sheets for repositioning patients. The pilot concluded with adoption of a superior chux product from a new vendor. Introduction of the new "GeriChux" was presented to the Value Analysis Team (VAT). It received conditional approval. The skin team had to show improved prevalence rates and cost effectiveness. This was to be documented along with an implementation teaching plan and reported back to the committee. Upon completion of this process, the CNS and skin staff contacted the EVS director to remove geripads. A mechanism was adopted to have the new GeriChux placed with the same par level in the same spot on the linen carts. Additionally, CCU staff opted for availability of a heavy draw for positioning immobile patients. Other units opted for the lighter draw sheet if needed for positioning. Team members initiated their PEP teaching projects during the month of May and June 2006 on their units. Laminated descriptions of the different products with cost and how and where to obtain supplies was posted strategically for staff.

Check: The quarterly prevalence study done immediately after the pilot revealed a drop in CCU pressure ulcer prevalence from 17.39% the previous quarter to 10.7%. The CCU rates fell below the national benchmark for the first time. Prevalence rates in the month of June 2006 were below the California Nursing Outcomes Coalition (CalNOC) Database Project benchmark at Palomar and on the POM medical surgical unit. The cost of linen dropped from the previous month and was below budget for the month of June 2006 in the geripad removal units.

Pressure Ulcer Prevalence:

Quality Report Cards Inform Staff Nurses About Pressure Ulcer Rates and Document Success of Quality Improvement Initiatives

115

NDNQI Data-Stimulated Practice Improvements Plans to Reduce Pressure Ulcers

Janet Hanley
Director, Critical Care
Janet.Hanley@sharp.com

Sharp Grossmont Hospital—LaMesa, California

Editors' pick:

INSIGHTS & IDEAS FROM THIS FACILITY

Cost of data collection is much smaller than the cost of pressure ulcers. Wound rounds and staff education were critical.

Facility Summary

Facility	Sharp Grossmont Hospital—LaMesa, California http://www.sharp.com/hospital/
Facility setting	Serves 750 square miles in east region of San Diego County. Acute care facility offering all inpatient and outpatient services including pediatrics, cancer center, hyperbarics, catheterization lab; 3,100 employees, 1,000 volunteers, more than 600 physicians, and 24,000 patient care admissions per year.
Teaching status	Non-teaching
Ownership status	Nonprofit organization
Community demographics	Community population growth expected to be 5.6% by 2007, 15.7% between the ages of 45 and 64 years, 76% Caucasian with the trend toward multicultural growth. Average household income for the east county region in 2004 was $66,439
Number of hospital staffed beds	457
Indicators used	Hospital acquired pressure ulcers, fall incidence, and staffing indicators related to both quality indicators
System or unit improved	System-wide across all nursing units
Indicator(s) improved	Hospital acquired pressure ulcers
QI report card/ document used	Monthly nursing report cards and NDNQI quarterly reports
NDNQI participant since	2004
Magnet™ status	Magnet designation received October 2006

UNIT PROFILE

Unit size and type	• Four progressive care units: two 41-bed units, 34-bed unit, and 19-bed unit • 41-bed surgical unit, 41-bed medical/oncology unit, 24-bed MICU, and 15-bed SICU
Unit RN staff profile	• Registered nurses, nursing assistants, unit clerks, and telemetry technicians in area of telemetry monitoring. • Medical–surgical units, RNs: 60% Associates, 34% bachelor's, 7% diploma or master's • Progressive care units RNs: 55% Associates, 41% bachelor's, 4% diploma or master's • Intensive care units RNs: 42% Associates, 54% bachelor's, 4% diploma or master's
Skill mix of RNs, other personnel	65–70% RN, 30-35% NA, MT,UC
Organizational structure of unit	Units have a director over the level of care, a manager, and lead/charge nurses (shift supervisors).

NDNQI Data-Stimulated Practice Improvements Plans to Reduce Pressure Ulcers

Janet Hanley
Director, Critical Care
Janet.Hanley@sharp.com

Introductory Summary:
HAPUs and Quality at Sharp Grossmont

Since 1999, Sharp Grossmont Hospital (SGH) has routinely collected statistics regarding pressure ulcers. This collection was done through chart audits and reports made to the wound team. However, an organized effort was lacking and a national benchmark was needed with which to compare hospital performance. Participation in the National Database for Nursing Quality Indicators (NDNQI) program provided opportunities to solidify and organize the SGH performance improvement process and to have access to a large database to provide comparisons.

To support organizational decision-making, performance results were systematically aggregated, statistically analyzed, and evaluated against targets on a regular basis. SGH committed to a data-driven performance improvement using the Six Sigma approach throughout the healthcare system in order to emphasize the importance of management using data to make decisions and to drive improvement efforts,. The "Voice of the Customer," rigorous process measurement, and statistical analyses are the cornerstones of Six Sigma, resulting in effective improvement strategies.

This approach provides Sharp Grossmont Hospital with strengths to build on:

- An evidence-based, measurement-focused aim to reduce excess and redundancy and improve consistency in processes and outcomes,

- A model that allows flexibility in the rigor of data analysis depending on the scope and complexity of the process and improvement tools used,

- A means to improve and manage the process to hold the gains, and

- A dedicated, multidisciplinary team of experts in the concepts of Six Sigma.

Quality reporting components (hospital-wide nursing practice council, Six Sigma projects, and other performance improvement teams) are hospital committees and departments that regularly report quality improvement initiatives progress and results to the SGH quality council. As members of the quality council, the CNO and other nursing leaders (director, emergency services; director, acute care services; director, critical care services; director, women's services; director, surgical services; director, rehabilitation services; and manager, behavioral health services) are responsible for presenting nurse-sensitive indicator results and other nursing-related improvement initiative outcomes to the interdisciplinary membership.

Introductory Summary:
Facility at a Glance

Sharp Grossmont Hospital, a 481-bed medical campus is the only nonprofit hospital serving San Diego's east county. The hospital is focused on providing patient-centered care, innovative technologies, and the most advanced medical treatments available while maintaining the staff and facilities to accommodate a growing community. Established on the principle of excellence, SGH provides services for emergency and basic trauma, acute care, cardiovascular, cancer care, neurological, stroke and neurosurgical, women's and children's, surgery, orthopedics, rehabilitation, behavioral health, and outpatient care.

The community served by Grossmont Healthcare District is approximately 750 square miles. Approximately 5% of the population that is served by SGH lives in remote or rural areas of this region. To service the community, SGH has over 3,100 employees, 1,000 volunteers, and more than 600 physicians and allied health professionals to provide care to over 24,600 patients admitted to the hospital (FY 2005). The population of the east county region is estimated at 466,000 people, or approximately 16% of the total San Diego County population.

Introductory Summary:
Unit Staff Profile

Several units have participated in the NDNQI data collection for skill mix, falls, and pressure ulcer prevalence indicators since Q1-04. The units include a 41-bed medical-oncology unit, a 41-bed surgical unit, four progressive care units with a total of 135 beds, a 24-bed medical intensive care unit, and a 15-bed surgical intensive care unit. As of Q4-05, the 30-bed acute rehabilitation unit formally joined the data collection process.

Each unit is staffed by registered nurses, nursing assistants, unit clerks, and telemetry technicians in the area of telemetry monitoring. Associate-degree nurses comprise nearly 60% of the RN staff on the medical surgical units, while 34% are BSN-prepared. Diploma and master's-prepared nurses make up 7%. In the progressive care units, 55% of the nurses have Associate degrees, 41% have bachelor's degrees, and 4% have a diploma or a master's degree. In the intensive care units, 42% of the nurses have associate degrees, 54% have bachelor's degrees and 4% have either a diploma or master's degree.

The acute care units are staffed at a ratio of one registered nurse to four to five patients. The progressive care units are staffed one registered nurse for every three to four patients, and the intensive care units are staffed at a ratio of one nurse to either one or two patients. All units are staffed based on the acuity level of the patients and the activity in the units. Each unit has a charge nurse for each shift and a manager responsible for the day-to-day operations.

NDNQI Startup Considerations

Participation in the NDNQI database began shortly after SGH's participation in a state database, the California Nurses Outcome Coalition (CalNOC), in late 2003. The SGH leadership team acknowledged the importance of formally collecting these data and benchmarking both at a state level and throughout the United States and determined the process for data collection and requirements. We knew that such a process would need to be set up to refine our data collection phase.

While there were costs, in both time and money, associated with the quarterly prevalence studies, data entry, and analysis of the results, they were found to be minimal when compared to the cost of treating a significant hospital-acquired pressure ulcer. Although work had started on both pressure ulcer issues and fall incidence, we believed that NDNQI participation would provide a broader data comparison on a national level and the ability to share best practices. One of the guiding principles of our nursing service is the drive for continuous quality improvement using data to seek improved outcomes.

Quality Measurement and Reporting

The director of critical care at SGH became the site coordinator for the NDNQI reporting process. Working closely with the chief nurse officer and the director of quality improvement, a system was established for data collection, communication of results, action plans for improvement, and celebration of wins and monitoring of progress.

Patient care requires a foundation built on knowledge-driven care practices. Evidence-based nursing care uses valid and reliable data and the ability to assess performance against nationally recognized databases. SGH developed its nursing report card to focus on quality, demographic, financial, and human resource areas. The monthly report aggregates unit-specific data to assist the nursing staff in evaluating trends and improving performance. Data elements important to nursing services were integrated into the report, including a set of nurse-sensitive indicators related to patient falls, skin, and medication practices. The nurs-

ing report card is shared on multiple levels throughout the organization. The report card is used for budget planning, unit goal development, and educational needs assessment purposes, and is routinely shared with bedside staff, physicians, leadership, and board members.

In order to ensure effective data utilization, several key processes have been implemented:

- The first step was to engage direct care nurses in the data collection process by offering educational presentations to prepare them as data collectors.

- The next step was to establish key communication linkages to the council structure. The nursing leadership council and the hospital-wide nursing practice council (HWNPC) ensure the dissemination of information to all direct care nurses to enable unit feedback.

- The nursing report card was refined to include pressure ulcer data.

- An indicator of hospital-acquired pressure ulcer prevalence was added to the annual evaluation of each employee on the nursing units.

Unit representatives are responsible for sharing information with colleagues and, in return, providing feedback from the direct care nurses and staff to the councils.

Through these mechanisms, the HWNPC and nursing leadership have been able to more actively engage the voices of staff in each practice setting and reshape the practice environment at SGH. Managers also receive the NDNQI fall and skin reports each quarter. An analysis is completed of the individual unit results and opportunities for celebration or improvement are discussed with the director. In 2005, the quality director added the NDNQI indicators to the hospital overall report card for discussion at both quality council and board meetings.

Quality Improvement of Hospital-Acquired Pressure Ulcers

In 2004, our initial data reflected a 17.69% HAPU rate in intensive care, a 13.95% HAPU rate in progressive care, and a 5.17% HAPU rate in acute care. These results were not expected. Immediately, nursing leadership took ownership of the results. The results were shared with staff in each individual unit and their unit practice councils were asked to develop a performance improvement project. The unit practice councils, made up of a cross-section of direct care nurses and other unit staff, worked with the wound team on improvement strategies:

- The first step was to update our guidelines of care for the prevention and treatment of pressure ulcers. Education was provided to the bedside staff and physicians about wound prevention, immediate identification of current and future skin issues, and evidence-based treatment. Additionally, the wound liaison role was created and staff volunteered to be the wound resource nurses on each unit. Research was shared that reflected the cost of treating a HAPU ranges from $4,000 to more than $70,000.

- The next step was to develop wound rounds (similar in format to a prevalence study) three times per week on each unit. This approach complemented the training previously established to better identify potential or actual skin issues on admission. The wound rounds included nursing leadership, staff, and the wound resource nurses.

- Action plans, which included who, what, and when, were developed to address even the slightest increase in HAPU. These action plans addressed why the pressure ulcer occurred, what education needed to be done, and who was the responsible party to correct the problem. All action plans, such as re-education of the nursing assistants, were acted on immediately and monitored frequently. During the next prevalence study, the action plan was addressed again to make sure the issues were resolved.

The process was refined over time after each quarterly report. Individual performance standards related to skin care were incorporated into the performance evaluation system of the staff and management.

Nursing staff, physicians, and leadership were very favorably impressed with the sustained improvement with the decrease in hospital-acquired pressure ulcers. This indicated that the hard work put into this initiative was working. Our patients were receiving the highest quality of care and we were successful in driving down costs. Our results have been celebrated throughout the hospital. The Q1-06 HAPU rate in intensive care was 0%, while our rate in 2004 was 17.70%. The progressive care units averaged 2.01% in Q1-06, while our rate in 2004 was 13.95%, and our acute care units averaged 2.74% in Q1-06, compared with our 2004 rate of 5.17%. Figure 1 illustrates these changes.

Each unit has celebrated its successful results. These favorable results were also noted in annual evaluations of staff and management. Staff have presented these results in local conferences and within our own organization.

Lessons Learned

Insights gained over our first years that have strengthened the program include:

- Support for the program at all levels of the organization,

- Taking ownership of the data and results by bedside staff and leadership,

- Invaluable expertise of the wound team,

- Creating the role of the wound liaison nurse on each unit,

- Making changes last through the key roles of education and follow-up,

- Thinking outside the box and celebrating your wins,

- Being willing to take time to make the change a permanent part of each unit's culture,

- Continuously monitoring the progress towards success, and

- Addressing issues immediately.

Conclusions and Implications

Prior to join NDNQI, we did not have national benchmarking abilities. With our first set of results, we realized the magnitude of SGH's challenge with hospital-acquired pressure ulcers. We have been able to develop an action plan, based on continuation of generating and using NDNQI's reliable data, that has resulted in excellent improvements in our patient care, increased strategies for prevention, identification, and treatment of pressure ulcers. We also found that this resulted in increased satisfaction among staff, physicians, and patients.

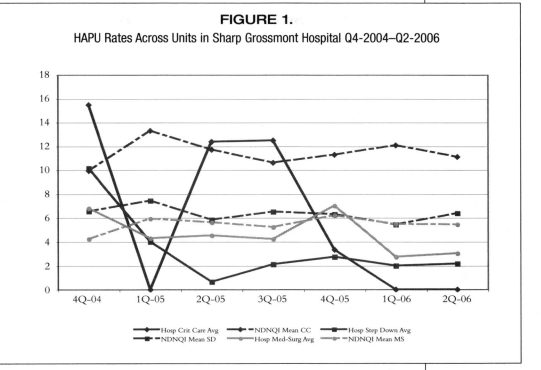

FIGURE 1.

HAPU Rates Across Units in Sharp Grossmont Hospital Q4-2004–Q2-2006

We will continue to work with our data each quarter and improve our program as needed. With each quarter's results, we assess what needs to change, what we need to expand on, what education has to take place, and where we need to next direct our attention. The HAPU prevalence indicator will continue to be a measurement point on performance evaluations for staff and management.

Pain Assessment/ Intervention/ Reassessment Cycle

Defined:

Pain Assessment—a comprehensive evaluation of pain location, characteristics, onset/duration, frequency, quality, intensity/severity and precipitating factors. It includes observation of behavioral and physiologic signs of discomfort, especially in those unable to communicate. Assessment is conducted using a valid and reliable, age-appropriate instrument. The tool selected is at the discretion of the participating institution.

Pain Intervention—the selection and implementation of a variety of measures (e.g. pharmacologic, nonpharmacologic, interpersonal) to facilitate pain relief (Nursing Intervention Classification, 2000). The administration of sedatives or hypnotics without analgesia is not considered a pain intervention.

Pain Reassessment—the subsequent evaluation of the effectiveness of pain relief measures following the intervention(s). The reassessment must fall within the time frame for intervention reassessment as defined by the unit/hospital standards.

Complete Cycle—*A complete pain assessment/intervention/reassessment cycle* is the documentation in the medical record of all three components of pain management listed above conducted by the professional nurse caring for the patient.

Formula:

Number of documented complete pain cycles/total number of cycles reported

Rapid Cycle Performance Teams Use NDNQI Data in Balanced Score Card to Improve Pain Management in Children

Georgeann Hall, MSN, RNC, CNA
Patient Care Manager, 4th and 6th Med–Surg
ghall@chsomaha.org

Judy Timmons, MSN, RN
Inpatient Clinical Nurse Specialist

Kristin Hopwood, BSN, RN, CPN
Clinical Nurse Coordinator, 4th Med–Surg

Pamela Ridder, BSN, RN, CPN
Staff Nurse, 4th Med–Surg

Kim Teaford, BSN, RN, CPN
Clinical Nurse Coordinator, 4th Med–Surg

Pamela Johnson-Carlson, MSN, RN, CAN
Director of Inpatient Services

Dena Belfiore, MSN, RN, CHRM
Vice President of Quality and Outcomes

Children's Hospital—Omaha, Nebraska

Editors' pick:

INSIGHTS & IDEAS FROM THIS FACILITY

Recognized elements of organizational change, highlighted for staff their direct impact on patient outcomes, and changed patient documentation systems. Each nurse now receives a report card.

Facility Summary

Facility	Children's Hospital, Omaha—Nebraska **www.chsomaha.org**
Facility setting	Only pediatric hospital in an area serving Nebraska, southwest Iowa, and parts of Kansas, Missouri, and South Dakota. Patients referred region-wide for complex or unusual disease treatment in addition to pediatric primary care. In addition to general pediatrics, offers numerous specialty services including newborn intensive care, pediatric critical care, and pediatric emergency services. Regionally distinctive services include 24/7 in-house services by pediatric critical care specialists and the state's only pediatric emergency department. ECMO services and a 24/7 neonatal/infant transport team for a 150-mile radius of Omaha. One of the nation's only eating disorders programs that accepts children as young as age five; provides inpatient, outpatient, and partial day services.
Teaching status	Primary inpatient teaching site for the joint Creighton University–University of Nebraska pediatric residency program. Also the pediatric training site for the family practice residency programs for many of the region's nursing and health professions schools and colleges.
Ownership status	Independent, nonprofit healthcare facility guided by a group of community leaders who serve on the board of directors.
Community demographics	Urban setting within metropolitan Omaha, covering eight counties in two states. Population of the Omaha Metropolitan Service Area is 807,305 with 85% of residents being white, 7.4% black or African American, 2.2% Asian, and less than 1% of several other races. Residents with Hispanic ethnicity approximately 6% of the population. Between 1990 and 2000, the population grew by approximately 12%, with growth to slow to approximately 5% between the 2005 and 2010. 30% of population under the age of 20.
Number of hospital staffed beds	142

Unit size and type	24-bed pediatric med–surg unit, primarily for newborns to 18 months
Indicators used	Pain assessment, intervention, response cycle documentation
System or unit improved	4th Med–Surg
Indicator(s) improved	Pain assessment, intervention, response cycle documentation
QI report card/ document used	Pain management is one of the metrics on the organizational balanced scorecard.
NDNQI participant since	2005
Magnet™ status	Children's Hospital received Magnet designation in December 2006.

UNIT PROFILE

Unit RN staff profile	43 RNs: RNs with professional nursing certification—17; Level of RN education—1 MSN, 30 BSN, 8 ADN, 4 diploma. Years of nursing experience at Children's averages 5.4 years, with a range of 6 weeks to 27 years.
Skill mix of RNs, other personnel	67% of direct care is provided by the RN staff and 0.17% of direct care is provided by LPNs. Child care partners in the assistive technician role provided 32% of direct patient care.
Organizational structure of unit	Direct care staff report to their assigned house supervisory clinical nurse coordinator (CNC), who is responsible for efficient operational flow of the area during the shift. The house dupervisory CNCs report to the patient care manager (PCM), who is responsible for the day to day operations of the unit. The director of inpatient services has overall accountability and responsibility for the operations and continuous improvement activities. Chief operating officer/chief nursing officer provides executive leadership for hospital operations (including division of nursing) for organizational and departmental strategic goals and objectives.

Pain Assessment/Intervention/Reassessment Cycle:
Rapid Cycle Performance Teams Use NDNQI Data in Balanced Score Card to Improve Pain Management in Children

131

Rapid Cycle Performance Teams Use NDNQI Data in Balanced Score Card to Improve Pain Management in Children

Georgeann Hall, MSN, RNC, CNA

Judy Timmons, MSN, RN

Kristin Hopwood, BSN, RN, CPN

Pamela Ridder, BSN, RN, CPN

Kim Teaford, BSN, RN, CPN

Pamela Johnson-Carlson, MSN, RN, CAN

Dena Belfiore, MSN, RN, CHRM

Introductory Summary: Quality Improvement at Children's

Driven by its mission, "so that all children may have a better chance to live," Children's Hospital in Omaha, Nebraska, was an early adopter of rapid-cycle performance improvement initiatives. Rapid-cycle performance improvement is an ongoing process that defines objectives for new services to assure a child-friendly delivery system. Process maps and flow charts are used to confirm value added steps in system design. Performance is compared to that of other pediatric organizations to seek best practice in selected areas. Data are continuously analyzed at all levels of the system, selecting areas for priority attention. The rapid-cycle improvement process utilizes brainstorming and pilot project processes when safety and quality must be enhanced. The model used for performance improvement activity is Plan, Do, Check/Study, Act (often shortened to PDSA).

Beginning its NDNQI participation in Q2–2005, Children's chose the two pediatric nursing practices benchmarks, pain management and peripheral IV infiltrations. Children's experience to date with the NDNQI pain management data and its related pain assessment/ intervention/response (AIR) cycle tool is the basis for this profile. After only three quarters, the pediatric medical–surgical unit profiled here achieved 100% compliance with the pain AIR cycles, and is maintaining that level of compliance.

The leadership team is responsible for developing and communicating the vision for quality and safety, then building organization-wide commitment to its achievement. The vision is deployed through the development of a plan for quality and patient safety. All levels of employees actively participate in improvement activities, allowing us to live our mission and achieve our vision.

Pain Assessment/Intervention/Reassessment Cycle:

Teams and councils of employees studying our facility's improvement opportunities are key to maintaining our safety and quality culture. Individual team members are motivated by their desire to provide safe, efficient evidence based care to our children.

A balanced scorecard is used to keep staff informed of important performance metrics. This scorecard clearly identifies important measures and targets. It provides a holistic view of the quality and safety of performance which strives to provide real-time data. The balanced scorecard moves us beyond *what* is being done to *how well* things are being done. Rapid-cycle performance teams, use of pilot projects and a balanced scorecard to convey outcomes are three of the distinctive ways Children's promotes its culture for quality and safety.

Introductory Summary: Facility at a Glance

Children's Hospital is a 142-bed independent non-profit healthcare facility under the direction of a dedicated group of community leaders who serve on the Board of Directors. The hospital employs nearly 1,800 dedicated staff. Patients are referred from throughout the region for the treatment of complex or unusual diseases in addition to pediatric primary care. The hospital serves as the primary inpatient teaching site for the joint Creighton University–University of Nebraska pediatric residency program. Children's also serves as the pediatric training site for the family practice residency programs at Clarkson Hospital, Creighton University, and University of Nebraska. The hospital supports 8 nursing schools in the region and 21 other schools for allied health professions.

Children's Hospital achieved the American Nurse's Credentialing Center's Magnet Recognition award on December 20, 2006.

NDNQI Startup Considerations

In the organization's pursuit of Magnet recognition, the decision was made to participate in the NDNQI database starting with Q2–2005. Pain management and peripheral IV practices were chosen as these were the only pediatric nursing benchmarks available at the time. Direct care nurses from all units who are members of our house-wide Clinical Practice Council (CPC) endorsed the idea of participating in NDNQI. These nurses felt it was important to be able to compare organizational nursing care practice with other pediatric inpatient settings. Clinical Practice Council members determined that they would collect and analyze the NDNQI data at the monthly council meetings. Time was allocated for this "field work" where the direct care nurses on the council evaluated clinical activities of their peers using the NDNQI prescribed pain management data collection tool.

Each quarter since, CPC members have analyzed the NDNQI pain management data results. With this analysis, CPC members evaluated the current policy and procedure on pain management to make sure appropriate standards of care that are reflected in the content. When the pain management policy/procedure was confirmed, CPC members identified that data from Q2–2005 demonstrated all inpatient areas had achieved higher rates of pain assessment/intervention/response (AIR) cycle documentation than one particular unit. These data confirmed that high levels of pain AIR cycle documentation were obtainable. CPC members recommended that the Area Action Council (AAC), namely, the 4th Medical–Surgical unit, become actively involved in further data analysis for their unit to develop an action plan.

4th Med–Surg is a 24-bed unit that focuses primarily on patients who are newborn to 18 months of age. This general unit cares for patients with both medical and surgical needs, along with other sub-specialties such as oncology, gastroenterology, endocrinology, neurology, pulmonology, and infectious diseases. In Q3–2005, the unit was composed of a staff of 62, including 1 Patient Care Manager (PCM), 4 House Supervisory Clinical Nurse Coordinators (CNC), 1 Clinical Nurse Educator, 32 Staff Nurses, 21 Child Care Partners and 3 Receptionists. Eleven nurses had achieved Certified Pediatric Nurse (CPN) status as of September 2005.

An average of 67% of direct care was provided by the RN staff. Child care partners in the assistive technician role provided 32% of direct patient care and 0.17% of direct care was provided by LPNs. The direct care staff report to their assigned House Supervisory CNC, who is responsible for efficient operational flow during the shift. The House Supervisory CNCs report to the PCM, who is responsible for the day to day operations of the unit. The director of inpatient services has overall accountability and responsibility for the operations and continuous improvement activities of this area. The chief operating officer/chief nursing officer provides executive leadership for hospital operations including the division of nursing in order to accomplish organizational and departmental strategic goals and objectives.

The Area Action Council is a work group composed of direct care nurses from both shifts and unit nursing leadership who come together for a monthly meeting. As part of our shared governance system, each unit's AAC is actively involved in problem solving unit issues related to clinical care, the work environment, and professionalism. In 2005, 4th and 6th Med–Surg nurses collaborated on a combined AAC as their unit processes were similar.

Quality Measurement and Reporting

Children's Hospital uses a balanced scorecard as a method to report aggregate quality data. Scorecard data include measures of personnel resources needed to support hospital business, care management, organizational growth, financial resources, service to customers, and select measures related to quality patient outcomes. These select measures of quality are chosen for their

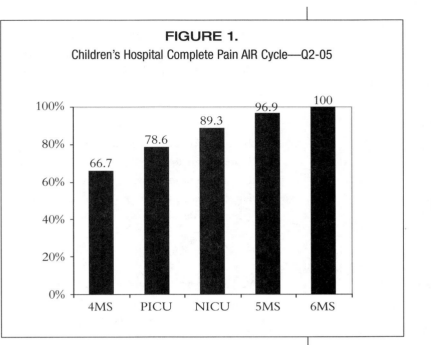

FIGURE 1.
Children's Hospital Complete Pain AIR Cycle—Q2-05

far-reaching impact on major patient populations or those indicators that have an opportunity for significant improvement.

In 2005, the organization used a global balanced scorecard as a tool for the senior leadership team and Board of Directors to use in evaluating systems and process for overall organizational effectiveness. As a result of the organization's entry into the NDNQI system in second quarter 2005, the Board of Directors approved the addition of Pain AIR cycle management documentation as a 2006 indicator for quality patient outcomes. In 2007, each patient care area is developing a unit-specific balanced scorecard to provide a mechanism for the area to maintain an ongoing pulse on their quality achievements and opportunities for improvement.

Quality Improvement of Indicator

When Q2–2005 NDNQI data were presented to the 4th/6th Med–Surg AAC, the data demonstrated nursing documentation of a complete pain AIR cycle on the day of audit was 66.67% of the time (Figure 1). The nurses were motivated by these results, since it was obvious that other units in the organization were able to achieve appropriate pain AIR cycle documentation. This AAC worked to develop a plan that would improve their practice and ultimately improve patient care on the unit. The AAC members evaluated nursing knowledge, pain AIR cycle documentation education, systems, and processes that supported this nursing practice. Evaluation of these steps identified several factors that contributed to inconsistency in practice, including knowledge deficit, education, and systems parameters, all of which are detailed below.

Knowledge Deficit

- AAC members identified a knowledge deficit among their peers about the use of the N-PASS pain assessment tool for infants in Med–Surg and not just those infants cared for in the NICU.

- Nurses and child care partners (nursing assistants) collaborate on providing patient care on 4th Med Surg. There was confusion among the nursing staff as to the child care partner's role in reporting the patient's pain when the child care partner obtained vital signs.

- Parents' perception of their infant's pain largely drove the nurse's administration of pain medications. This was challenging for some nurses as the nurse's pain assessment using a standardized pain assessment tool did not always indicate that the child was in pain. The nurse had to synthesize the conflicting assessment information to make a plan for pain management.

Education

- New employee orientation is a critical time for new nurses to gain appropriate new skills. The AAC group confirmed that the orientation process for new nurses to understand pain management was appropriate and included the required elements. They identified that preceptors needed to repeatedly emphasize each component of the pain AIR process and how to document it appropriately. With ongo-

ing emphasis on pain AIR cycle documentation throughout orientation, the orientee would develop a strong habit for documentation. In addition, an ongoing component of orientation included a meeting with the orientee, preceptor, unit educator, and unit manager to discuss progress toward the completion of orientation.

- Nurses had received education on pain AIR cycle documentation several times in the past year. Staff nurses had identified that at times it was difficult to assimilate information due to the rapid rate of change. 4th Med–Surg nurses requested ongoing education reminders to keep changes in practice in the forefront.

Systems

- All Med–Surg units converted to a new patient documentation flowsheet in May 2005. Prior to the implementation of this new flowsheet, 4th Med–Surg nurses were charting an infant's pain as generalized pain, when the codes for documentation did not include generalized pain. Documentation processes were unclear and did not match the requirements for documentation. In addition, pain documentation had been scattered throughout the Med–Surg patient flowsheet, which created confusion for nurses. Nurses would at times make up their own way of charting because there were too many places to document on the flowsheet. In general, nurses had a sense that their documentation of pain was not always complete and there were many complaints of duplication of charting and a cumbersome process.

- The AAC members identified that a learning curve for use of the new Med–Surg patient flowsheet could influence the accuracy pain documentation. The group's first action step was to evaluate the newly implemented (May 2005) Med–Surg flowsheet to confirm that it would facilitate consistent documentation of pain management and alleviate duplication of charting as pain documentation was consolidated into one location.

Based on these parameters, the 4th/6th AAC members evaluated the newly implemented Med–Surg flowsheet to confirm that it facilitated consistent documentation of pain AIR cycle information and duplication was reduced.

Ongoing education for the nursing staff was another priority strategy developed by AAC. This included providing a blitz of information about pain assessment scales, interventions, and reassessment of pain. Methods included providing education through multiple means. At change of shift report, the CNCs reminded the nurses on shift to improve their pain AIR cycle documentation. A newsletter called the "Newsreel" was emailed to all nurses with clarifications on how to use the infant pain assessment tool; reminders to complete pain AIR; and resources to use if the nurse was unsure about some aspect of pain management. An example from the April 2005 Newsreel stated:

"Newsreel Topic #17—
Pain Documentation on new Flow Sheets

- *When you give a medication as an intervention for pain, you only have to document the fact that a med was given. (i.e. an "m" in the intervention column). You do not have to document what medication it was—that information is in the MAR.*

- *Remember to check the type of pain assessment tool you will be using most often. If you assess pain using another tool, you are to put an ★ in the tool column and then write in the exception notes that a different tool was used."*

Another strategy included providing short focused education highlights in the staff restroom, called "Learning in the Loo," which addressed identified learning needs. Education in a fun, creative method caught people's attention and provided an easy reminder of specific pain AIR cycle documentation.

An addition was made to the nursing orientation process. Regular conferences were held with a new orientee, the preceptor, the clinical educator, and the PCM to discuss progress toward the achievement of required competencies and the completion of nursing orientation. With the 4th Med–Surg NDNQI pain AIR cycle results, a new focus in this discussion related to the orientee's understanding of pain AIR cycle documentation.

Most importantly, the AAC members identified that real-time learning would yield results. Staff nurses reported that they understood the pain AIR cycle documentation in theory, but would find challenges in documenting individual situations. In response, the House Supervisory CNCs completed chart audits on each 4th floor patient's discharged chart using the NDNQI pain assessment tool. The information was used as an opportunity to mentor individual nurses on how to improve their pain AIR cycle documentation. The House Supervisory CNC and the staff nurse discussed the challenges the nurse had in documenting the pain AIR cycle information and clarified misconceptions.

The results of these combined efforts were very positive as a significant improvement in pain AIR cycle documentation was noted. A sustained improvement has been seen as 100% compliance has been maintained through Q1–2006 (Figure 2).

Lessons Learned

Lessons learned were multifold. The quality of data collection tools is important to obtaining quality results for interpretation. We noted the Performance Improvement department collected data on pain AIR cycle documentation using a different data collection tool than the NDNQI tool. This meant that we had two different types of pain AIR cycle data to analyze with conflicting results. The decision was made to use the NDNQI data collection tool for consistent

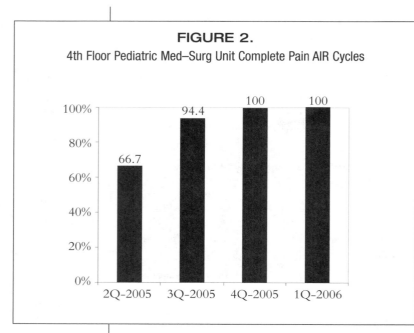

FIGURE 2.
4th Floor Pediatric Med–Surg Unit Complete Pain AIR Cycles

measurement in the organization which yielded comparable results. The NDNQI Pain AIR cycle assessment tool ensured that we could obtain results that we trusted as it had been previously validated. Internal inter-rater reliability in data collection was an issue. Each time data on pain AIR cycle documentation were collected, CPC spent time reviewing the data collection tool and clarifying the points of data collection before the nurses completed their "field work" to obtain the data.

While repeated education and clarification of practice are important, the most significant impact was seen when the individual nurse's performance was highlighted. When staff nurses heard reports of NDNQI pain AIR-cycle documentation data at their staff meetings, they stated that they felt that their performance had no impact on the results as they didn't make mistakes. When the House Supervisory CNC met with individuals on their poor performance in documentation, she approached the nurse with the intent that a knowledge deficit was the contributing factor to the nurse's poor documentation. When the staff nurse noted that her supervisor was positively invested in her performance and misconceptions were clarified, the nurse understood that her performance did influence overall unit performance. The nurse became more

motivated to improving her performance. Costs for this process were limited as the mentoring took place while the nurse was on shift. Effective change can be made when aggregate data is drilled down to the individual practitioner.

Conclusions and Implications

For 2006, pain management has become an indicator of overall organizational performance. The House Supervisory CNCs on each unit continue to audit discharged patient records and provide ongoing mentoring with the direct care staff nurses on their performance related to pain AIR-cycle documentation. CPC continues to collect pain AIR-cycle documentation data for the quarterly NDNQI report. The combined results of these audits are aggregated and presented to the Senior Leadership Team in their monthly Balanced Scorecard Results.

In the future, each nurse will receive a quarterly report card with her individual results related to pain AIR-cycle documentation. The individual nurse results will be blinded and posted in aggregate in each unit as an additional personal motivator for nurses to compare their performance against their peers. As the nurses continue to see where individual performance influences total unit performance on quality indicators, it is hoped that they will remain motivated to incorporate changes related to performance improvement activities into their daily practice.

In conclusion, pain management will always be a priority for nursing practice as nurses continue to strive toward a higher level of understanding of effective pain assessment, intervention and re-evaluation. As a result of this priority focus, a positive effect on patient outcomes may be seen as patients and their families develop greater trust in the nursing staff to effectively manage their pain. In a trusting relationship, the patient, family, and nurse can collaborate on the aspects of care that will promote healing and the patient's more expedient return to home..

RN Satisfaction

The *NDNQI RN Satisfaction Survey* contains the NDNQI adaptation of Stamps' (1997) *Index of Work Satisfaction* (adapted with permission of Dr. Paula Stamps). Stamps defines job satisfaction as "the extent to which people like their jobs" (p. 13), and "views it as a complex, multidimensional construct that captures individual's reactions to specific components of their work" (Taunton, et al, 2004, p. 102). The *NDNQI-Adapted Index of Work Satisfaction* subscales are defined below:

- Task: Activities that must be done as a regular part of the job

- Nurse-Nurse Interactions: Formal and informal contact among nurses during working hours

- Nurse-Physician Interactions: Formal and informal contact with physicians during working hours

- Decision-making: Management policies and practices related to decision-making

- Autonomy: Amount of independence, initiative, and freedom permitted or required in daily work activities

- Professional Status: Importance or significance of the job, both in nurses' and others' view

- Pay: Cash remuneration and fringe benefits received for work performed

Also included are the NDNQI® adaptation of selected items of the Aiken and Patrician (2000) *Revised Nursing Work Index* (adapted with permission of Dr. Linda Aiken). Aiken and Patrician developed this instrument as an organizational environment measure. The *NDNQI-Adapted Nursing Work Index* subscales are defined below:

- Professional Development: Opportunity and access to career development

- Supportive Nursing Management: Satisfaction with unit managers in relation to decision, support, and consultation

- Nursing Administration: The visibility and power of the chief nursing officer.

The Job Enjoyment scale, which was developed from Brayfield and Rothe's (1951) questionnaire, is defined as follows:

- Job Enjoyment: Measure of the degree to which people like their work

Aiken, L. & Patrician, P.A. (2000). Measuring organizational traits of hospitals: The Revised Nursing Work Index. *Nursing Research, 49,* 146-153.

Brayfield, A. & Rothe, H. (1951). An index of job satisfaction. *Journal of Applied Psychology, 35,* 307-311.

Stamps, P. (1997). *Nurses and work satisfaction: An index for measurement.* Chicago: Health Administration Press.

Taunton, R.L., Bott, M.J., Koehn, M.L., Miller, P., Rindner, E., Pace, K., Elliott, C., Bradley, K.J., Boyle, D., & Dunton, N. (2004). The NDNQI-Adapted Index of Work Satisfaction. *Journal of Nursing Measurement, 12,* 101-122.

Using Results from the NDNQI RN Satisfaction Survey to Improve Satisfaction and Patient Outcomes

Thelma Gray-Becknell, RN, MSN
Chief Nursed Executive

Lottie Lockett, RN, MS, CNAA, BC
Associate Chief Nurse

Molly Alex, RN, MSN, CAN, BC
Nurse Manager

MaryAnne Reese, RN, MSN
Staff Nurse

Michael E. DeBakey Veterans Affairs Medical Center—Houston, TX

Editors' pick:

INSIGHTS & IDEAS FROM THIS FACILITY

Examined certain components of satisfaction, worked to improve them, and addressed scale scores at staff meeting discussions.

Facility Summary

Facility	Michael E. DeBakey Veterans Affairs Medical Center—Houston, TX http://www.houston.med.va.gov/
Facility setting	Urban-based quaternary care, facility providing comprehensive inpatient and outpatient care in medicine, surgery, mental health, spinal cord injury, physical medicine and rehabilitation, neurology, audiology, speech pathology, ophthalmology, long-term care, and home care. Primary health care provider for more than 116,000 veterans in southeast Texas. Veterans from around the country are referred to center for specialized healthcare services. Also operates four outpatient clinics in Beaumont, Lufkin, Galveston, and Texas City.
Teaching status	Teaching, with the largest VA residency program in the United States
Ownership status	U.S. Department of Veterans Affairs, Veterans Health Administration
Community demographics	Urban, rural, and suburban mix
Number of hospital staffed beds	343 hospital beds; also a 40-bed spinal cord injury center and a 120-bed transitional care unit for long-term care patients.
Indicators used	Patient falls, pressure ulcer prevalence, nursing hours per patient day, skill mix, and RN satisfaction
System or unit improved	Nursing Unit 4D
Indicator(s) improved	RN satisfaction
QI report card/ document used	Unit score card
NDNQI participant since	July 2003
Magnet™ status	Awarded in August 2004

UNIT PROFILE

Unit size and type	Nursing Unit 4D—Step-down unit; intermediate care and geriatric patients with a bed capacity of 25 (one of 20 MEDVAMC inpatient units of similar size).
Unit staff profile and skill mix of RNs, other personnel	A nurse manager oversees 12 RNs, 8 licensed vocational nurses, 5 nursing assistants, and a program support assistant. Also on the interdisciplinary team are a social worker, two physician assistants, and a physician as the unit administrator who provides administrative guidance and medical care.
Organizational structure of unit	Nursing unit 4D is in the extended care line at the medical center and an RN serves as the care line executive.

Using Results from the NDNQI RN Satisfaction Survey to Improve Satisfaction and Patient Outcomes

Thelma Gray-Becknell, RN, MSN
Chief Nursed Executive

Lottie Lockett, RN, MS, CNAA, BC
Associate Chief Nurse

Molly Alex, RN, MSN, CAN, BC
Nurse Manager

MaryAnne Reese, RN, MSN
Staff Nurse

Introductory Summary

Satisfied staff nurses are less likely to leave their jobs, resulting in a reduction of recruitment efforts for facilities and lower turnover rates (Shader K, Broome ME, Broome CD, West ME, & Nash M, 2001). The National Database of Nursing Quality Indicators (NDNQI) creates and makes available to its members an annual RN satisfaction survey. This survey serves to ensure nursing management has concrete evidence supporting their nurses' satisfaction level on the job. The staff on nursing Unit 4D at the Michael E. DeBakey Veterans Affairs Medical Center (MEDVAMC) indicated in their 2004 submission for this survey overall moderate satisfaction[1] (2004) scores associated with the 10 subscales of the nursing work index and the job enjoyment scale. Repeating the same survey one year later, the RNs indicated higher satisfaction levels in all of the categories measured. While all categories are measured at the unit level, a portion of the survey pinpoints the individual nurse, their concerns and feelings, in the 10 subscales of nursing work satisfaction items and the category of satisfied with my job. At the individual level, with one exception, Unit 4D showed great improvement year over year in all job satisfaction categories except one. This positive change in job satisfaction occurred after one full year of interven-

---

1. T-scores measurements--Low satisfaction <40; Moderate Satisfaction 40-60; High satisfaction >60

tion and much hard work to bridge gaps identified in the 2004 survey.

NDNQI's annual survey allows facilities to understand a variety of metrics as they relate to working relationships (i.e., peer-to-peer, doctor-to-nurse), organizational culture, and the satisfaction of nurses at one hospital compared to similar hospitals nationwide. The NDNQI survey is easily accessible online; therefore, nurses can choose to take the survey at work or at home. With a real-time administrative interface, nursing management is able to view the survey response rate at anytime during the 21-day survey process. While access to the nurses response rate is readily available, the names of nurses who have completed (or not completed) the surveys are confidential. This method facilitates open and honest comments regarding the various job satisfaction opportunities in the units and within the hospital at large. At the conclusion of the survey period, NDNQI provides a composite of the data collected as well as a benchmark of the specific hospital surveyed compared with other hospitals participating in NDNQI. Most Magnet-designated hospitals, or those seeking Magnet designation, join NDNQI and have the opportunity to participate in the annual RN satisfaction survey process.

In addition to the nurse staff satisfaction trends and benchmarks being a Magnet requirement, MEDVAMC fully supports the process because of the perspective it provides, and consequently participate in the NDNQI nurse satisfaction survy. This survey is particularly helpful in identifying target areas that, when appropriately addressed, potentially can increase nursing satisfaction. That, in turn, results in more consistent care because nurses are less likely to leave the facility or unit, thus increasing patient satisfaction. In exploring the results of the 2004 NDNQI job satisfaction survey, 4D nursing staff found the following issues drove down employee satisfaction: trust, team work, empowerment, responsibility, and confidence. All of these areas were considered dynamics linked to those concepts measured by the survey. To ensure complete team buy-in and participation in building a

more satisfying place to work, 4D nursing staff worked in tandem with management to implement a plan that appropriately identified their concerns and targeted realistic resolutions.

Facility at a Glance

MEDVAMC is a teaching hospital located in Houston, Texas, that operates the largest residency program in the U.S. Department of Veterans Affairs (VA) healthcare system. The medical center was awarded Magnet recognition for excellence in nursing service in 2004. The MEDVAMC serves as the primary healthcare provider for more than 112,000 veterans in southeast Texas. Locally, MEDVAMC is a part of the world renowned Texas medical center community where over 43 healthcare institutions are strategically positioned in the Houston metropolitan area. As a quaternary (beyond tertiary phase) medical center, MEDVAMC has 521 operating beds, with a classified Level 2 emergency room, four offsite clinics, and provides a full range of inpatient care and outpatient services. Organizationally, MEDVAMC is composed of care and service lines, and is governed by an oversight senior leadership team with care and service line executives.

The DeBakey medical center is one of the 163 hospitals in the VA's Veterans Health Administration. The typical unit in MEDVAMC consists of between 25 and 35 beds. Units are managed by nurse managers who oversee the various RNs, licensed vocational nurses, nursing assistants, and program support assistants. The level of staff working on a unit at any particular time varies based on the level of care required by the patients and the scope and complexity of the unit (i.e., acute, intermediate). Nursing is not the only healthcare component on a MEDVAMC unit. Most units are interdisciplinary, having one or more social workers, physician's assistants, and physicians. Working in tandem, the unit's healthcare professionals ensure the highest quality of care for the nation's military veterans located in southeast Texas.

MEDVAMC became a member and participant of NDNQI in July 2003 and adopted all of the nurse-sensitive indicators: patient falls, nursing hours per patient day, skill mix, pressure ulcer prevalence, and RN satisfaction. The RN satisfaction indicator allows participation by all units and clinics, some of which might otherwise not qualify to participate in data collection for other indicators. Beginning in 2004, MED-VAMC has conducted the RN satisfaction survey annually during the month of September. The participation of each of the 37 nursing inpatient units and clinics in the RN satisfaction indicator is vital to understanding the progress of the total facility in terms of overall job satisfaction. The composites received from NDNQI serve to highlight areas of strengths that can be leveraged throughout the various units and opportunities that provide a platform for growth and development among the nursing teams.

Unit Staff Profile

Nursing unit 4D, a combination of intermediate medicine and geriatric patients, is one of 20 inpatient units at the MEDVAMC with a bed capacity of 25. A nurse manager provides oversight for a skill mix of 12 RNs, 8 licensed vocational nurses, 5 nursing assistants, and one program support assistant. Other healthcare professionals who comprise the interdisciplinary team on 4D are one social worker, two physician assistants, and a physician who serves as unit administrator providing administrative guidance and medical care. Nursing Unit 4D resides organizationally in the extended care line, where a nurse serves as the care line executive, and provides what in most healthcare facilities is referred to as long-term care (Figure 1).

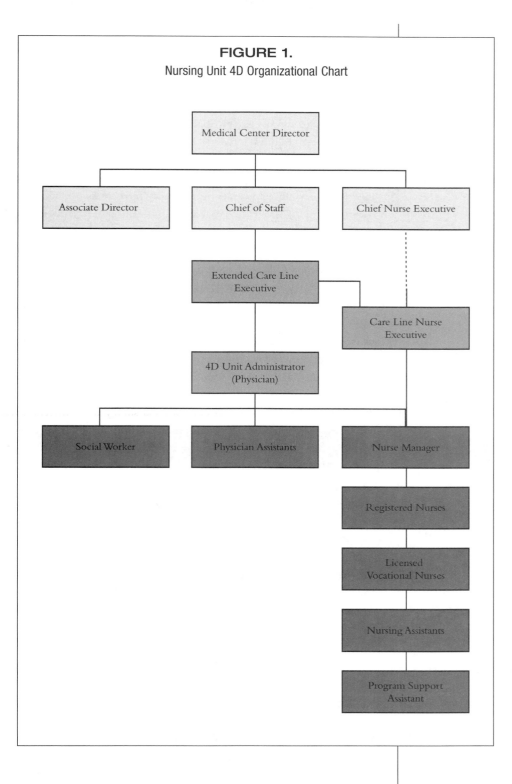

FIGURE 1.

Nursing Unit 4D Organizational Chart

Medical Center Director

Associate Director

Chief of Staff

Chief Nurse Executive

Extended Care Line Executive

Care Line Nurse Executive

4D Unit Administrator (Physician)

Social Worker

Physician Assistants

Nurse Manager

Registered Nurses

Licensed Vocational Nurses

Nursing Assistants

Program Support Assistant

NDNQI Startup Considerations

MEDVAMC began using NDNQI in summer 2003. All indicators were adopted and data collected for outcome measurements and benchmarking, which occurred in August 2003. Results of the nursing metrics received from the completed NDNQI indicator analyses provided valid and reliable measurements of current efforts and helped identify strategic target areas for improving MEDVAMC's results and the status quo.

MEDVAMC's first RN satisfaction survey was conducted in September 2004 with a hospital response rate of 90% and a 100% response rate on nursing unit 4D. Nursing Unit 4D embraced the RN satisfaction indicator with great enthusiasm. Nurses anonymously indicated levels of satisfaction with factors directly related to their jobs, tasks, values, and the essential qualities associated with the job. The nurses, led by the RN satisfaction "champion" (one of their peers on the unit), rallied together to achieve 100% participation within the first week that the RN satisfaction survey was administered. Nurses were awarded a $10 gift certificate to the MEDVAMC retail store for their participation. Nursing Unit 4D also achieved 100% participation in the RN satisfaction survey the following year.

MEDVAMC had previously been involved in another national database that measures nurse-sensitive indicators. This previous experience familiarized nurses with the indicator concept. In transitioning to the NDNQI system, only minor operational maneuvers required explanation and training. NDNQI, which provides a more comprehensive set of metrics, focused in more detail and thus provided a better perspective on critical issues at the hospital.

Quality Measurement and Reporting

The following figure illustrates a prototype of the unit score card[2] highlighting nursing Unit 4D and MEDVAMC's T-scores resulting from the RN satisfaction surveys in 2004 and 2005 (Table 1).

The unit score card is only one way to display and communicate results of the nurse-sensitive indicators. Graphs are also used to reflect a more interpretable summary of the T-scores and serve as a quick reference point for needed improvement. The official web-based report received from NDNQI is sent to all nursing leaders.

The nursing quality circle at MEDVAMC, an open interactive forum, was created to disseminate data-driven results to staff, like the NDNQI survey results. The chief nurse executive provides feedback to the executive council, made up of the senior management and the care and service line executives. Senior managers communicate to their nurse managers. Nurse managers review, identify, and discuss opportunities for improvement during their unit meetings. The nursing web page under construction will serve as a tool for displaying nurse-sensitive indicator data for the medical center.

Quality Improvement

In reviewing the composites for the 4D unit, the nurse manager identified issues driving down the satisfaction of registered nurses on the unit. In the survey, 4D nurses outlined tasks, team work, and decision-making, as issues dragging down workplace satisfaction. As the problems revolved around basic empowerment and team issues, the focus of process improvement was readily evident.

The RNs articulated their feeling related to team work on the unit. A majority of the nurses were performing many of the nurse assistants' tasks, while struggling to complete their own work. The nursing assistants appeared to have excessive free time, even though work had been delegated and assigned to them. Conflicts among the unit's personnel were a daily occurrence. The group was not working as a team. In overcoming

---

2. Unit score card is used for displaying data for various measures at the unit level.

these obstacles, the first step was for staff members to share concerns and clearly articulate and resolve differences regarding the approach to patient care and unit management. The nurse manager initiated a team meeting to define the opportunity and work needed to ensure positive change. As the staff became engaged, application of the FOCUS-PDSA[3] model evolved. Once the FOCUS-PDSA performance improvement model was implemented, the metrics related to the various index scales in the RN

TABLE 1.

Unit 4D's Nurse-Sensitive Indicator Unit Score Card: RN Satisfaction Survey Results from the NDNQI-Adapted Index of Work Satisfaction Scales

Subscales	Unit T-Scores 2004	MEDVAMC 2004	Unit T-Scores 2005	MEDVAMC 2005
Tasks	**43.83**	**46.03**	*50.27*	46.75
RN–RN	**52.29**	**63.96**	*69.07*	**63.35**
RN–MD	60.72	69.02	*71.59*	62.08
Decision-making	50.26	49.01	*59.88*	**48.61**
Autonomy	52.21	**48.99**	*62.55*	**48.03**
Professional status	66.77	67.78	*79.84*	67.40
Pay	51.08	44.70	*51.96*	45.79
Professional development	**60.88**	**60.11**	*76.89*	**61.01**
Nursing management	**55.48**	57.82	*67.80*	59.45
Nursing administration	57.88	58.60	*67.29*	57.54
Job enjoyment	**53.46**	55.66	*69.60*	55.65

T-scores are listed above with the following values: <40 = Low satisfaction ... 40–60 = Moderate satisfaction ... >60 = High satisfaction ... *Italic* indicates values above national scores... **Bold** indicates below national scores.

satisfaction survey revealed by NDNQI were highlighted and used as a yardstick to note those traits or lack of traits identified by the staff. For example:

Traits Identified by Staff on 4D	Index Items of NDNQI
Empowerment	Autonomy
Critical Thinking	Decision-making
Assignment/Documentation	Task
Team Work	RN–RN Interaction

The first and most important attribute the staff needed to redefine as a team was trust. Trust is built by working collaboratively and successfully interacting with one another. Staff adapted the following "mantra" indicating the type of unit they strove to become: "Be strong, but not rude. Be kind, but not timid. Be bold, but not a bully. Be proud, but not arrogant. Be humorous without folly and deal in realities." (Rohn 2003)

The nurses reapplied the art of delegation and regained confidence in making decisions. According to Stricklin

(2006), delegation creates job satisfaction and promotes team work. Therefore, emphasis was given on how to delegate as licensed professionals and hold each person responsible for their assignment. A 4D unit council was established to: strengthen and promote autonomy; share accountability for unit operations; communicate ideas, concerns, and needs; and identify and resolve unit-level issues of practice, quality, professional development, and work environment.

The team's sense of empowerment and team work was evident in the 2005 annual NDNQI RN satisfaction survey when the T-scores for job enjoyment rose to 69.60 – over 16 points above the prior year (Figure 2). The T-scores related to job satisfaction also rose to 74.75—up over 17 points (Figure 3). Both of these scores represented significant progress and improve-

---

3. FOCUS-PDSA is the performance improvement methodology model used at MEDVAMC. F=Find; O=Organize; C=Clarify; U=Understand; S=Study; P=Plan; D=Do; S=Study; and A=Act.

FIGURE 2.

Chart of RN Job Satisfaction T-Scores—Selected Individual-level Item Results for 2004 and 2005

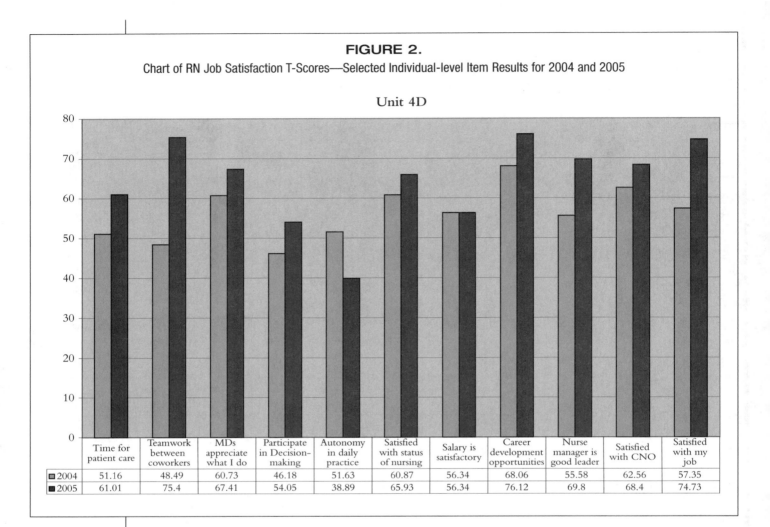

Unit 4D

	Time for patient care	Teamwork between coworkers	MDs appreciate what I do	Participate in Decision-making	Autonomy in daily practice	Satisfied with status of nursing	Salary is satisfactory	Career development opportunities	Nurse manager is good leader	Satisfied with CNO	Satisfied with my job
▪ 2004	51.16	48.49	60.73	46.18	51.63	60.87	56.34	68.06	55.58	62.56	57.35
▪ 2005	61.01	75.4	67.41	54.05	38.89	65.93	56.34	76.12	69.8	68.4	74.73

ment in the unit, but the most significant change was the nurses' desire to remain on the unit. In the 2005 survey, 100% of the nurses said they desired to remain on the unit over the next year, a significant improvement over the 43% who indicated a desire to remain on the unit the previous year. The impact was most evident in the turnover and absentee rate for the unit. The unit's turnover rate dropped from 6.27% in 2005 to 1.33% in 2006 and absenteeism decreased from 9.57% in 2005 to 4.37% in 2006. Patient outcomes also improved. The fall rate dropped by greater than 50%, from 57% in 2005 to 23% in 2006. Medication errors decreased from a total of 11 med errors in 2005 to zero in 2006. Documentation has also improved in 2006 with 100% compliance on both PRN effective-

ness and pain assessment. Satisfied nurses make tough decisions when needed and produce positive patient outcomes.

One unsettling negative trend was in the individual-focused work index item associated with autonomy in daily practice. This T-score decreased from 51.63 in 2004 to a low of 38.89 in 2005 (Figure 2). When autonomy was measured for the unit and group, the nurses' T-score level rose from 52.21 in 2004 to 62.55 in 2005. This shift seemed peculiar and completely contrary to the work put forth by the unit. While this was not a desired outcome, it did serve the total team well and facilitated the changes necessary to increase total satisfaction.

Lessons Learned

Following the NDNQI 2005 annual RN Survey, the nurses on 4D highlighted the obvious changes in T-scores and applauded the efforts of all, not just particular individuals. It was very clear that the common denominator that stimulated satisfaction among the nurses on nursing Unit 4D was the team concept and how the team functioned or did not function as a unit. Usually, people want to do the right thing and do the right thing right. When a team is not performing effectively, it is perhaps because an element of job dissatisfaction exists among the team members. Listed below are the lessons learned from nursing unit 4D, which reflect attributes of the team after a common direction was determined:

- A cohesive team builds and promotes positive attributions in the work environment with positive outcomes.

- Team members are empowered and energized when they address issues and concerns in a positive, constructive way.

Conclusions and Implications

The NDNQI RN survey provides an invaluable gauge of RNs' perception of the numerous traits that influence the scale, either positively or negatively, for measuring job satisfaction. Utilization of the survey tool affords the nurses on nursing Unit 4D the opportunity to honestly express, without negative consequences, the perceptions and feelings of how satisfied they are with their jobs.

As illustrated in 2004, nurses on nursing Unit 4D scored in many categories at a level unacceptable to them as a team. Having participated in the NDNQI survey, they were able to face the challenge and explore options as well as set in motion alternatives to improve their situation. Without the NDNQI survey data, the satisfaction of the nurses on nursing 4D would have probably continued undefined, since the hard evidence-based data needed to institute the positive change would not have been available.

The annual NDNQI RN survey provides a built-in mechanism to: identify issues to target on individuals unit and facility-wide; target job enhancement opportunities; capture feedback from the point of care staff; and benchmark with other healthcare facilities of comparable complexity.

References

Rohn, J. (2003). Jim Rohn's Weekly E-zine. Issue 215. December 16.

Shader K., Broome M.E., Broome C.D., West M.E., and Nash M. (2001) Factors influencing satisfaction and anticipating turnover for nurses in an academic medical center. *Journal of Nursing Administration* (4):210–6. April 31.

Stricklin, R. (2006). Learning to delegate in the clinical setting. http://www.nurse.com/Nurse Content/Community/NurseCommentary/Delegating.htm.

Job Enjoyment as an Indicator of Successful Shared Governance

Arlene J. Costello, MS, RN CNAA-BC
Director, Maternal Child Nursing

Patricia Kurz, MPS, CEN, CMSRN, CNA-BC
Director, Medical–Surgical Nursing
patricia.kurz@chsli.org

Good Samaritan Hospital Medical Center—West Islip, New York

Editors' pick:

INSIGHTS & IDEAS FROM THIS FACILITY

Demonstrated clear linkage when satisfaction increased, so did patient outcomes. Recognized the importance of the night shift.

Facility Summary

Facility	Good Samaritan Hospital Medical Center—West Islip, New York http://goodsamaritan.chsli.org/
Facility setting	Services include ambulatory surgery, pain management, birth place with more than 3,000 deliveries per year, and high-risk obstetrical service including Level 3 neonatal intensive care unit and pediatric intensive care unit. Also have an outpatient Center for Pediatric Specialty Care with comprehensive pediatric services in cardiology, neurology, pulmonary, endocrinology, hematology, gastroenterology, and infant/child development.
	The oncology and radiation oncology services have been recognized by the Commission on Cancer and the American College of Surgeons as offering the highest quality cancer care. The palliative care department includes an acute palliative care unit.
	New York State Department of Health designation as a stroke venter in 2005.
	Level 2 trauma center in emergency department with 85,000 visits per year and the only dedicated pediatric emergency department on the south shore of Long Island, New York.
	Primary angioplasty program within the cardiology department. Acute and chronic dialysis services and a full range of diagnostic and imaging services. Comprehensive inpatient and outpatient rehabilitation services, as well as medical–surgical and critical care nursing services.
Teaching status	Affiliation with New York College of Osteopathic Medicine and offers residency programs in family practice, pediatrics, obstetrics, and emergency medicine.
	Clinical rotations are provided for approximately 600 nursing students in four BSN and two AAS programs.
Ownership status	Nonprofit community hospital
Community demographics	Suburban setting with a service area population of 813,011 and an average household income of $85,966. The population is predominantly white (79.8%), with continued growth in the Hispanic (7.2%) and African American (9.3%) populations.

Number of hospital staffed beds	431
Indicators used	Job enjoyment
System or unit improved	System-wide
Indicator(s) improved	Job enjoyment
QI report card/ document used	Departmental and unit-based report cards
Magnet™ status	October 2006

Job Enjoyment as an Indicator of Successful Shared Governance

Arlene J. Costello, MS, RN CNAA-BC
Director, Maternal Child Nursing

Patricia Kurz, MPS, CEN, CMSRN, CNA-BC
Director, Medical–Surgical Nursing

Introductory Summary

The success story of the Department of Nursing at Good Samaritan Hospital Medical Center (GSHMC) is one of transformation from a centralized management structure to one of decentralized staff empowerment and engagement.

Quality improvement activities had been addressed historically as predominantly process related studies. Most of these activities were completed by the management team with little or no contribution (beyond data collection) from the bedside staff. In 2003, as a result of JCAHO's influence on staffing effectiveness studies using nurse-sensitive indicators, the focus changed to outcome-driven indicators

Prior to 2003, RN satisfaction was neither measured nor prioritized. The nurses at the bedside had little control over decisions affecting their practice. The arrival of a new CNO in the fall of 2002 brought with it a new vision for a decentralized shared governance model, improved patient outcomes and heightened staff satisfaction. The rising RN vacancy rate provided an added incentive to introduce change.

NDNQI Startup Considerations

Recognizing that a focused plan would be necessary before embarking on this journey, the leadership team, led by the new CNO, prepared a strategic plan early in 2003. Strengths and weaknesses of the existing structure were discussed candidly. Managers were provided the education and tools they needed to reach new heights in accountability and outcomes.

Bolstered by our Magnet journey, which began shortly thereafter, profound changes were made in the structure and culture of the Department of Nursing. The

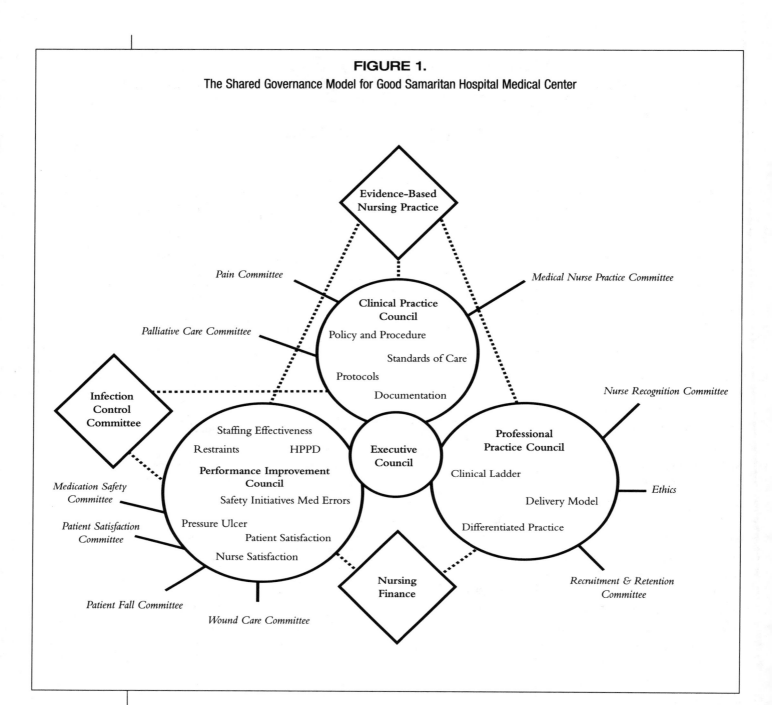

once centralized management structure was transformed into one of shared governance that put the bedside nurse at the decision-making body and made the Nurse Manager effectively the CEO of the unit. The model of this organizational transformation is shown in Figure 1.

Quality Measurement and Reporting

While evidence-based, nurse-sensitive indicators were chosen to measure clinical excellence, the NDNQI RN Satisfaction survey was used to measure the success of the new governance model. Initially distrustful of the survey, the staff needed to be gently coaxed into participation. The shared governance model was yet in its infancy and the 2003 RN Satisfaction Survey results were envisioned as the starting point in the Magnet Journey. This was confirmed by the wide gap between the GSHMC 2003 job enjoyment score and the "NDNQI Hospitals" score. The NDNQI Hospital scores reflect voluntary participation by 131 U.S. hospitals of all sizes (from fewer than 100 to more than 500 beds) that participated in the survey in 2003. This sample represented 2,943 nursing units, which equalled 41,524 RNs.

The Nurse Managers took the 2003 data back to the bedside staff and developed unit-specific strategic plans to increase RN satisfaction. Most of the units identified and addressed issues that would ultimately reinforce the development of the shared governance model.

Progress was slow as the 2004 job enjoyment scores indicate. Not only had the 2003 score fallen even lower, the gap between GSHMC and the other hospitals had widened. We thought that this initial decrease in satisfaction resulted from high response rates from RNs who chose not to join in the Magnet journey. The establishment of a shared governance model is traditionally a five year journey (Porter-O'Grady, 2005). The work done in 2003 and 2004—to lay a foundation for shared governance—began to bear fruit in 2005. This was demonstrated by a sharp rise in the GSHMC job enjoyment

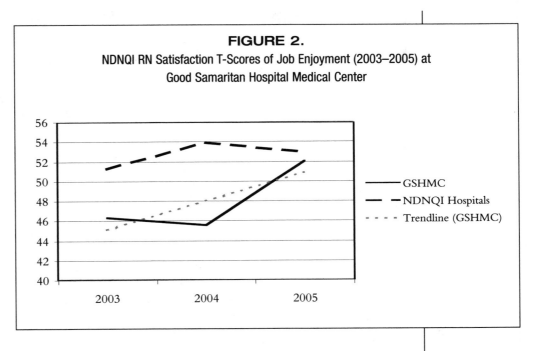

FIGURE 2.
NDNQI RN Satisfaction T-Scores of Job Enjoyment (2003–2005) at Good Samaritan Hospital Medical Center

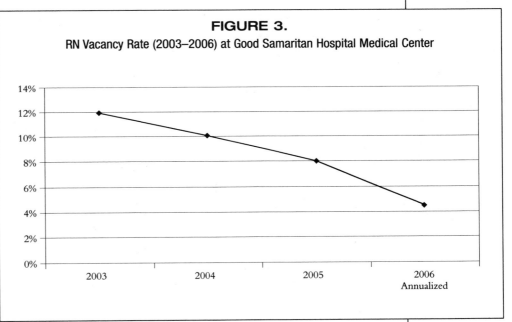

FIGURE 3.
RN Vacancy Rate (2003–2006) at Good Samaritan Hospital Medical Center

scores, accompanied by a significantly narrowed margin between GSHMC and the other hospitals. See Figure 2 for a representation of these three years of scores

Since the NDNQI RN satisfaction data are available only annually, another indicator was sought to measure satisfaction on a more frequent basis. RN vacancy

TABLE 1.

RN Vacancy Rate at Good Samaritan Hospital Medical Center

			GSHMC Vacancy Rates			
Indicator	Definition	Benchmark	2004	2005	Q1–06	Q2–06
HUMAN RESOURCE INDICATORS						
RN Vacancy Rate	Three-month average of vacant RN FTEs divided by three-month average total number of RN FTEs	10.0%	10.07%	8.00%	4.00%	5.00%

Source: Average 2004 Vacancy and Turnover Rates for Registered Nurses. Hospital Association of New York State Workforce Advocacy Survey Results; April 2005.

TABLE 2.

RN Job Satisfaction T-Scores at Good Samaritan Hospital Medical Center (GSHMC)

RN SATISFACTION Individual Level Items	GSHMC Data	National Comparison Data		
RN Job Satisfaction	2004	2003	2004	2005
Time for patient care	54.99	46.45	47.96	52.65
Teamwork between coworkers	70.73	69.75	65.91	71.48
Physicians appreciate what I do	61.02	54.57	53.03	59.87
Participate in decision-making	48.42	42.09	44.20	51.18
Autonomy in daily practice	50.04	45.52	43.53	48.69
Satisfied with status of nursing	54.41	41.53	44.10	52.34
Salary is satisfactory	51.33	40.04	42.57	48.82
Satisfied with my job	63.33	55.00	53.30	60.19
Career development opportunities	60.02	ND	53.71	64.83

Source: RN Satisfaction Survey (2004) Group—All units in all hospitals. National Database of Nursing Quality Indicators (NDNQI).

Quarterly RN Vacancy rates were added to the unit report cards and to the Executive Dashboard Report in addition to the NDNQI annual data. Nursing staff, as well as the managers, became well versed in the indicators and their ability to effect change in the values. As the job enjoyment score rose and the vacancy rate dropped, most of the remaining NDNQI scores rose. See Tables 1 and 2 for more details on these changes.

Lessons Learned

The successful implementation of the shared governance model ultimately led to GSHMC 2006 achievement of Magnet designation. It is impossible to put a price tag on that accomplishment. However, it is possible to do a cost–benefit analysis related to the decrease in the RN vacancy rate.

Based on industry estimates that it costs approximately $60,000 to replace one RN (Jones, 2005), the decrease in the RN vacancy rate from 10.07 % in 2004 to 4.5% in 2006 represents a $1,576,200 savings over three

rates provided that snapshot. Mirroring national trends, the Good Samaritan 2003 composite RN vacancy rate was reported at a startling 11.92% with a few selected units reporting rates significantly higher (Figure 3). This indicator provided the Nurse Manager the opportunity to look at trends on a monthly basis and to react appropriately.

years. During that same period of time (2004 through 2006) the implementation of the shared governance model in conjunction with the Magnet journey cost $602,548. This total includes salaries ($315,900), administrative costs ($9,000), staff compensation for meetings ($27,648) and total miscellaneous costs for the Magnet journey ($250,000). The net result is a savings of $973,652.

As nursing at Good Samaritan progresses on the journey towards Shared Governance internal data on quality, safety, productivity and cost support that we are approaching or exceeding the national benchmarks for performance for almost every nurse-sensitive indicator. Based on this it seems reasonable to form several assumptions. At GSHMC,

- There is an association between nurse satisfaction and patient satisfaction.
- Teamwork, autonomy and career opportunities are important to our nurses.
- Challenged by performance outcomes, nurses will improve patient safety.
- As the vacancy rate decreases, the absentee rate decreases.

Conclusions and Implications

The success story at Good Samaritan Hospital Medical Center is only beginning. Achievement of Magnet status is a journey, not a destination. It is expected that RN satisfaction, specifically job enjoyment, will continue as an upward trend. The following activities have been prioritized as the next steps:

- The shared governance model will reach maturation in 2007 with the establishment of unit based councils.
- All major councils will be active on the night shift.
- Divisional Quality Improvement activities will continue to grow and include unit-specific Quality Accountability models and decentralized meetings.

References

Jones, CB (2005). The Cost of Nurse Turnover, Part 2. *Journal of Nursing Administration* 35, 41-49.

Porter-O, T (2005). Tim Porter-O. Retrieved November 7, 2006, from Implementing Shared Governance, Creating a Professional Organization Web site: http://www.topgassociates.com/SharedGovernance.htm

Enhancing Professional Work Environment Results in Higher RN Job Satisfaction

Kristine M. Leahy-Gross, RN, BSN
Data Analyst, Nursing and Patient Care Services
k.leahygross@hosp.wisc.edu

Susan M. Rees, RN, MS
Nursing Director, Nursing and Patient Care Services

University of Wisconsin Hospital and Clinics—Madison, Wisconsin

Editors' pick:

INSIGHTS & IDEAS FROM THIS FACILITY

Unit-level distribution of satisfaction data in easy-to-read format allowed staff nurses input to the nursing council structure, thus improving practice environment satisfaction.

Facility Summary

Facility	University of Wisconsin Hospital and Clinics—Madison, Wisconsin http://www.uwhealth.org/
Facility setting	Academic medical center serving south-central Wisconsin and beyond.
Teaching status	Teaching
Ownership status	Public agency
Community demographics	• Per capita income for area is the third highest in the state and is $5,000 above the national average (2003) data. Dane county wages are 10% of the state average. Affluent population base able to spend more on health care. • The area has a higher percentage of people with graduate or professional degrees than the rest of the US (11.3% vs. 6.4%) Highly educated population with better understanding of healthcare factors. • 66.6 % of the population 16 years old or older is in the age group of 25–59 years old compared to the US percentage of 62.2%; 16.2% of the area population is over 60 years old compared to the rest of the US at 21.4%. Younger population–different healthcare needs. • Regional centers for higher education, research and government.
Number of hospital staffed beds	472 staffed beds
Unit size and type	Sixty-six areas participated in the annual 2005 RN satisfaction survey. This included inpatient, operative, clinic, home health, dialysis, coordinated care/case management, ED, and transplant services.
Indicators used	• Work Groups—Job enjoyment, task, decision-making, autonomy • Individuals—Satisfied with my job, time for patient care, participate in decision-making, autonomy in daily practice
System or unit improved	RN satisfaction
Indicator(s) improved	RN satisfaction
NDNQI participant since	2003
Magnet™ status	Intend to apply

Enhancing Professional Work Environment Results in Higher RN Job Satisfaction

Kristine M. Leahy-Gross, RN, BSN
Data Analyst, Nursing and Patient Care Services
k.leahygross@hosp.wisc.edu

Susan M. Rees, RN, MS
Nursing Director, Nursing and Patient Care Services

Introductory Summary

The University of Wisconsin Hospital and Clinics (UWHC), located in Madison, is an academic medical center that was created by the Wisconsin legislature in 1924 and reorganized as a public authority in June 1996. UWHC is independent and nonprofit, receiving no state funding except Medicaid reimbursement.

In October 2003, the RN staff had their first opportunity to participate in the NDNQI RN Satisfaction Survey. At that time, there was not a nursing collaborative governance model in place. In fact, most of the nursing committees were primarily populated with nursing leadership. As our collaborative governance model was constructed, a nursing council structure was formed that insured a minimum of 50% participation from frontline direct care RN staff, as well as the implementation of individual unit councils populated entirely by frontline staff.

Facility At-a-Glance

In FY 2005, there were 22,507 inpatient admissions, 124,565 patient days, and 547,673 outpatient visits in the UWHC system, which offers a wide array of services and programs through specialty clinics and UW Hospital that are described below.

The critical care program area includes the Med Flight critical care air transport service and Children's Hospital Emergency Transport Ambulance. The program's onsite facilities include a fully equipped emergency room, Level I trauma center for both adult and pediatric care; burn unit, and intensive care units for pediatrics, cardiac, CT surgery, neuroscience, and medical.

UWHC serves the oncology population throughout the UW Comprehensive Cancer Center with six regional cancer centers throughout Wisconsin and northern Illinois. The UW Children's Hospital, a

60-bed pediatric hospital, is nationally known for treatment of children's lung diseases, cardiac surgery, and other pediatric specialties.

The organ transplant program at UWHC is one of the largest programs in the United States, with patient outcomes consistently cited among the best in the nation (www.ustransplant.org). The heart and vascular care program offers a comprehensive program of prevention, expert diagnosis, and treatment of the full spectrum of heart-related diseases.

The stroke center offers a thorough set of stroke studies or treatments. This includes testing of multiple surgical interventions, advance diagnostic imaging, medications, and therapeutic interventions for acute stroke and its after effects.

UWHC is in the initial stages of Magnet status application and has participated in quarterly data submission to NDNQI since January 2003. Since then, quarterly nurse-sensitive indicator data have been submitted on 23 inpatient units. Sixty-six areas participated in the annual 2005 RN satisfaction survey. This included inpatient, operative, clinic, home health, dialysis, coordinated care/case management, ED, and transplant services.

Nursing Staff Profile

UWHC has 536 licensed and 472 staffed beds (five adult intensive care units with 56 beds) and 85 outpatient clinics. The nursing and patient care services program has five clinical inpatient divisions. The percentage of RNs in the units' skill mix are included in parentheses below:

- *Surgical and psychiatric nursing*—Burn unit (95%); general surgery and trauma unit (71%); GYN/urology/ENT and plastics unit (71%); neurosurgery unit (64%); neurosurgery ICU (85%); orthopedics unit (68%), transplant unit (73%) and psychiatry unit (75%)

- *Medical nursing*—Family practice and forensics unit (67%); general clinical research unit (98%); general medicine and geriatrics unit (67%); hemodialysis unit; pulmonary and renal unit (69%); radiology nursing and rehabilitation units (68%); trauma life support center ICU (81%)

- *Heart and vascular care services*—Thoracic and cardiac surgery unit (74%); cardiology unit (82%); cardiology ICU (87%); heart and vascular progressive care unit (76%)

- *Pediatric nursing*—Pediatrics age 6 and over and hematology/oncology units (81%); pediatric ICU (94%); pediatrics infant and toddler age 5 and under (88%)

- *Oncology services*—Oncology unit (64%)

- *Operative services*—Inpatient OR; inpatient PACU; outpatient surgery center OR; outpatient surgery center PACU/FDS

- *Home health*

- *Coordinated care/Case management*

- *Ambulatory nursing*

- *Dialysis*

- *Emergency department*—*Med Flight*

- *Transplant services*

Quality Measurement and Reporting: UWHC Quality Monitoring Structure

The quality structure of the UWHC nursing and patient care services is based on interdisciplinary teams including physicians, case managers, clinical nurse managers, clinical nurse specialists, nurse clinicians, and other health professionals. The teams are formed throughout the inpatient service with crossover to include clinicians from ambulatory, operative, and home health services. These teams set standards of care and practice across settings for specific patient populations through critical pathway development. The teams carry out analysis of clinical and fiscal variances and patient satisfaction data.

Findings are used to change practice and alter critical pathways.

There are several quality teams focused on specific patient care needs: pain, wound and skin, hematology/oncology, and diabetes. The teams reflect membership from clinical and support staff throughout the hospital, clinics, operative services, home health services, and medical and nursing schools. The teams set standards of care and practice related to their respective clinical focus. In addition to setting standards, the team is responsible for performance improvement through monitoring practice and related patient outcomes. The teams are charged with developing proactive programs to be incorporated into critical pathways and into patient and family teaching guidelines. The teams educate staff to assure that practice programs are implemented to the standard. Lastly, teams evaluate the impact of clinical program changes on desired outcomes and alter practice accordingly.

Primary responsibilities of nursing unit and department activities related to performance improvement are carried out through the nursing council structure and include implementation of quality control monitoring of nursing and hospital service standards, review and analysis of patient and staff satisfaction data, monitoring of compliance with regulatory standards, and development of nursing specific quality monitoring studies. Patient satisfaction is monitored through the Press Ganey survey and information is shared with the interdisciplinary teams and unit/department councils. Changes in practice are instituted as warranted and outcomes monitored to determine the effectiveness of changes.

Quality Measurement and Reporting: Role of the Nursing Council Structure

There are nine collaborative governance nursing councils that make up the UWHC's nursing council structure. These include councils on nursing: quality, product evaluation and standardization, practice, research,

advancement and recognition, credentialing, education, informatics, and a council of unit chairpersons. In addition, each unit has a council that reviews quality data, makes suggestions for practice change, and identifies issues for study. The council structure was implemented in January 2005.

Quality Improvement: Using the RN Satisfaction Survey

UWHC began submission of nurse-sensitive data to NDNQI in January 2003. Since that time, we have participated in the annual RN satisfaction survey thus providing comparative data per unit and overall since 2003. In October 2003, when RNs took the survey for the first time, we created incentives to achieve a higher response rate. These incentives included a coupon to the hospital cafeteria or an ice cream coupon for offsite clinics. An additional incentive included a pizza party for those units that achieved a 100% response rate. In 2003, there was a response rate of 65%. In 2004, there was a 22% increase in the response rate to 79% and in 2005 the response rate increased 5% to 83%. In 2005, there were 1,479 eligible participating RNs and 1,222 RNs completed the satisfaction survey. Of the 66 units participating, 33 units achieved a 100% response rate. Eligible RNs included those that spend at least 50% of their time in direct patient care and have been employed on the unit a minimum of three months.

Staff responses to the RN satisfaction survey were generally positive. With the advent of the unit council structure in January 2005, these data were widely disseminated and presented to all the nursing councils, in particular, to the council of unit chairpersons. This council was directed to discuss these data among their unit-level councils. The unit-level councils openly discussed problems thus empowering staff to resolve problems and increase satisfaction.

A key to the success of RN satisfaction was the sharing of the information with staff. Each unit's data

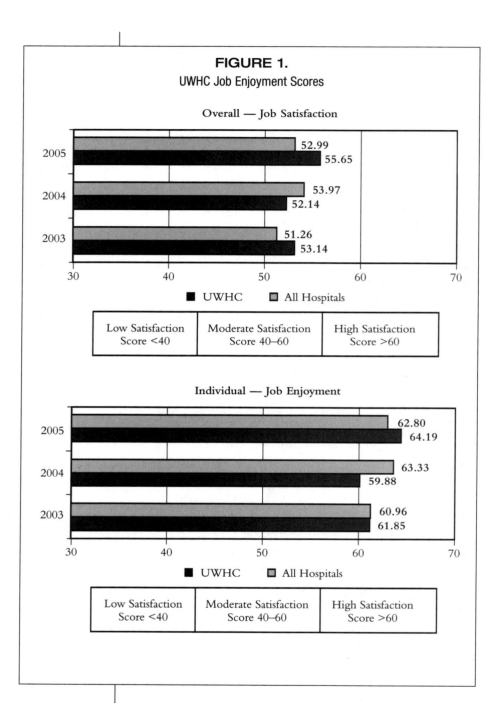

FIGURE 1.

UWHC Job Enjoyment Scores

Overall — Job Satisfaction

2005	52.99 / 55.65
2004	53.97 / 52.14
2003	51.26 / 53.14

■ UWHC ▨ All Hospitals

Low Satisfaction Score <40	Moderate Satisfaction Score 40–60	High Satisfaction Score >60

Individual — Job Enjoyment

2005	62.80 / 64.19
2004	63.33 / 59.88
2003	60.96 / 61.85

■ UWHC ▨ All Hospitals

Low Satisfaction Score <40	Moderate Satisfaction Score 40–60	High Satisfaction Score >60

The next few pages describe how four of the categories of survey data were applied and integrated into nursing practice over the course of three years. Job enjoyment, tasks, decision-making, and autonomy were selected because these areas showed substantial improvement from 2004 to 2005.

Quality Improvement: Applying the Job Enjoyment Scores

The nursing and patient care services staff at UWHC have celebrated many successes after more than three years of using the RN satisfaction survey and with a new senior vice president for patient care services and chief nurse officer (November 2003). The senior VP-CNO is visible to staff through weekly rounds on inpatient units and quarterly "coffee breaks" with staff. This informal break time with staff supports a culture of valuing staff and their feedback. The nurses see the CNO as being open and available. She has a positive impact on morale because of her habit of recognizing staff for even small achievements. The UWHC culture is shifting since the organization committed to achieving the goal of being the regional "employer of choice."

In an analysis on the impact of these organizational changes, the UWHC overall job satisfaction score in 2005 was found to be 55.65, which was 6.7% higher than 2004 (Figure 1). This score was statistically significantly greater than all hospitals and 5% greater than all hospitals in the NDNQI database. When considered on the basis of the individual employee, the 2005 job enjoyment score of UWHC RNs was 64.19 or 7.2% greater than 2004 (Figure 1). This score was statistically significantly greater than all hospitals, with UWHC having a 2.2% higher score.

were extracted from the NDNQI aggregate and graphed, allowing a display of each unit trend per category per year. By presenting these data in such an easy-to-read format, staff were able to readily understand the volume of data contained in the NDNQI report (Figure 1 on page 170).

Quality Improvement: Applying the Task Scores

UWHC implemented a professional practice model to provide a structure that better supports nurses. Primary nursing began with early adopter units in early 2005. This practice structure led to a more effective use of time through the continuity of patient care. Another factor leading to an increase in "task" nurse satisfaction was the RN hours per patient day. Generally, UWHC's RN hours per patient data results are higher than NDNQI mean for facilities with 400-499 beds. Hence, RNs at UWHC feel that they had enough time to complete the tasks that are needed for quality patient care.

At the overall level, UWHC RN's task score in 2005 was 49.61 or 7.6% higher than 2004 (Figure 2). This score was statistically significantly greater than all hospitals and 6.3% greater than all hospitals in NDNQI. When considered on the basis of the individual employee, the 2005 task score of UWHC RNs was 57.43 or 4.8% greater than 2004 (Figure 2). This score was statistically significantly greater than all hospitals, with UWHC having a 5% higher score.

Quality Improvement: Applying the Decision-making Scores

Clinical nurses participate in collaborative decision-making in many ways that include the nursing councils and focus groups. The focus groups, composed primarily of direct care staff, worked on complex issues such as narcotic administration and the nurse residency program. The unit council structure has also enhanced satisfaction with decision-making because unit staff are implementing change on their units.

At the overlall level, the decision-making score of UWHC RNs in 2005 was 45.65 or an 8.7% higher than 2004 (Figure 3). When considered on the basis of the individual employee, the 2005 score of UWHC RNs "participate in decision-making" was 47.56 or 10.3% greater than 2004 (Figure 3).

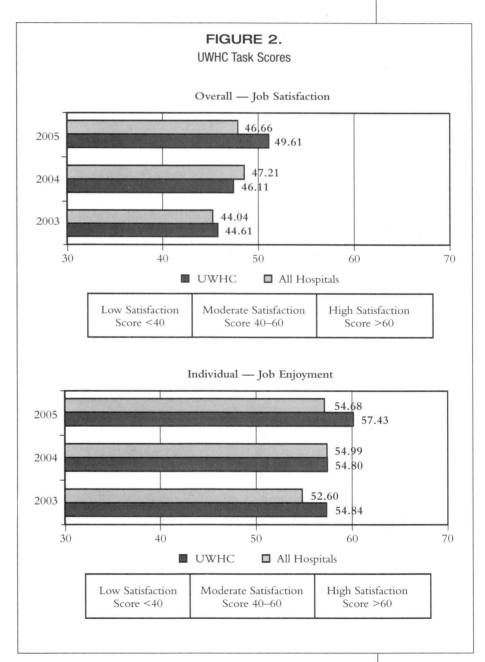

FIGURE 2.
UWHC Task Scores

Overall — Job Satisfaction

■ UWHC　□ All Hospitals

| Low Satisfaction Score <40 | Moderate Satisfaction Score 40–60 | High Satisfaction Score >60 |

Individual — Job Enjoyment

■ UWHC　□ All Hospitals

| Low Satisfaction Score <40 | Moderate Satisfaction Score 40–60 | High Satisfaction Score >60 |

Quality Improvement: Applying the Autonomy Scores

Primary nursing is designed to enhance the autonomy and responsibility of professional nurses. Along with the council structure, nurses' control over their practice is generally increasing. UWHC's unit council structure has been critical to increasing RN autonomy. The unit councils empower nursing staff to impact practice on their units. The primary nursing practice model enhances autonomy as well through independence within an interdisciplinary model of care. The collaborative governance council structure is changing the feeling of empowerment among nurses, as they are involved in decisions about nursing overall. There is continued focus on evidence-based practice, with a nursing research coordinator overseeing nursing research projects.

At the overall level, UWHC RNs autonomy score was 50.26 in 2005, or 8.8% higher than 2004 (Figure 4). When considered on the basis of the individual employee, the 2005 score of UWHC RNs in "autonomy in daily practice" was 50.9, or 3.2% greater than 2004 (Figure 4). This score was statistically significantly greater, with UWHC having a 2.9% higher score.

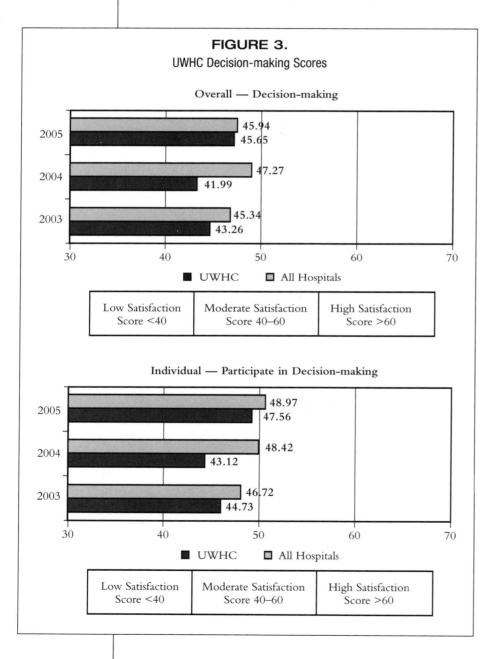

FIGURE 3.
UWHC Decision-making Scores

Overall — Decision-making

2005: UWHC 45.65, All Hospitals 45.94
2004: UWHC 41.99, All Hospitals 47.27
2003: UWHC 43.26, All Hospitals 45.34

■ UWHC ☐ All Hospitals

Low Satisfaction Score <40	Moderate Satisfaction Score 40–60	High Satisfaction Score >60

Individual — Participate in Decision-making

2005: UWHC 47.56, All Hospitals 48.97
2004: UWHC 43.12, All Hospitals 48.42
2003: UWHC 44.73, All Hospitals 46.72

■ UWHC ☐ All Hospitals

Low Satisfaction Score <40	Moderate Satisfaction Score 40–60	High Satisfaction Score >60

Lessons Learned

Our experience with improvements in RN satisfaction showed that data must be presented in a useful, functional way at the cost center level. The display of data at this level will promote a systematic approach to building upon a professional practice structure. In addition, the nursing council structure provides nursing staff input as well as a forum to encourage nursing satisfaction and to share results. The council structure gives nurses a voice and provides collegiality. The structure ensures the staff an opportunity to change things that are important to the unit. Staff are empowered through the council structure which leads to increased autonomy and improved RN satisfaction. We are continually improving the council structure and have recently implemented a co-chair for each nursing council. The councils are led by staff nurses and leadership representatives.

Conclusions and Implications

Using data such as those provided by the NDNQI RN Satisfaction Survey is a valuable way to encourage performance improvement among nursing staff that can lead to progress in professional nursing practice both at the unit and department levels. By sharing data with frontline staff and asking them to focus on improving in specific areas, this becomes a doable process. Having comparative data, both from other units within the organization and from other organizations, as well as trending the data over time, allows staff to see progress on the changes they have implemented to enhance their satisfaction. The NDNQI RN satisfaction survey also allows healthcare organizations to examine how changes within the department and throughout the organization impact RN satisfaction. In a time of nursing shortages, the imperative for keeping RN satisfaction levels high and continually trying to improve on it cannot be overlooked.

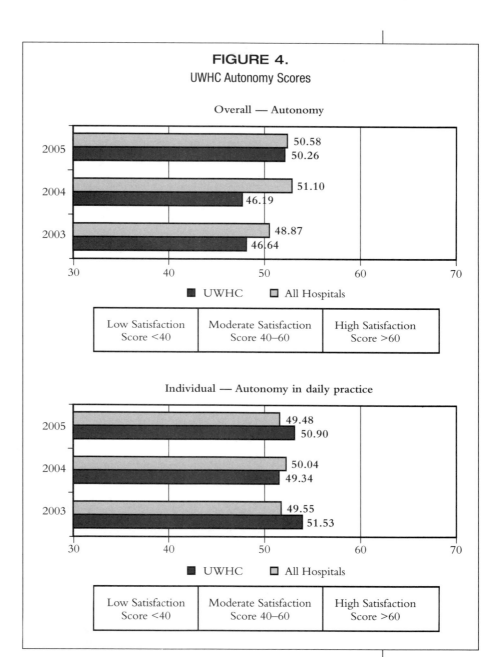

FIGURE 4.

UWHC Autonomy Scores

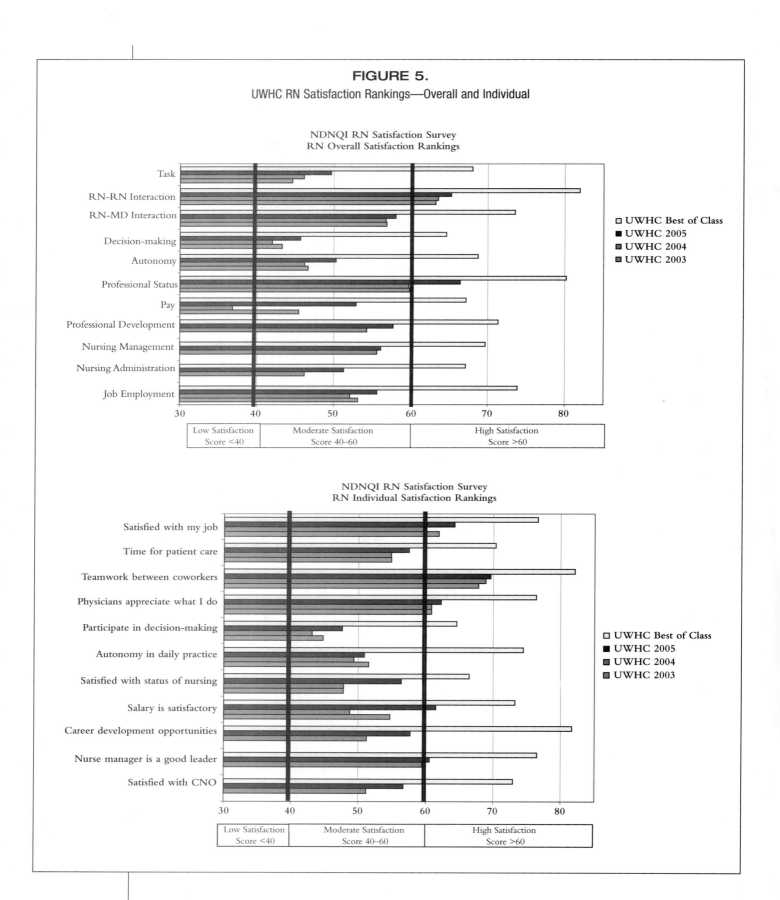

FIGURE 5.
UWHC RN Satisfaction Rankings—Overall and Individual

NDNQI RN Satisfaction Survey
RN Overall Satisfaction Rankings

Categories (top to bottom): Task, RN-RN Interaction, RN-MD Interaction, Decision-making, Autonomy, Professional Status, Pay, Professional Development, Nursing Management, Nursing Administration, Job Employment

Legend:
☐ UWHC Best of Class
■ UWHC 2005
■ UWHC 2004
■ UWHC 2003

| Low Satisfaction Score <40 | Moderate Satisfaction Score 40–60 | High Satisfaction Score >60 |

NDNQI RN Satisfaction Survey
RN Individual Satisfaction Rankings

Categories (top to bottom): Satisfied with my job, Time for patient care, Teamwork between coworkers, Physicians appreciate what I do, Participate in decision-making, Autonomy in daily practice, Satisfied with status of nursing, Salary is satisfactory, Career development opportunities, Nurse manager is a good leader, Satisfied with CNO

Legend:
☐ UWHC Best of Class
■ UWHC 2005
■ UWHC 2004
■ UWHC 2003

| Low Satisfaction Score <40 | Moderate Satisfaction Score 40–60 | High Satisfaction Score >60 |

Transforming Nursing Data Into Quality Care:
Profiles of Quality Improvement in U.S. Healthcare Facilities

Appendix A.
National Database
of Nursing Quality
Indicators[1]

Indicators[2,3]

- Nursing Hours per Patient Day★
  - Registered Nurses (RN)
  - Licensed Practical/Vocational Nurses (LPN/LVN)
  - Unlicensed Assistive (UAP)
- Patient Falls★
- Patient Falls with Injury★
  - Injury Level
- Pediatric Pain Assessment, Intervention, Reassessment (AIR) Cycle
- Pediatric Peripheral Intravenous Infiltration Rate
- Pressure Ulcer Prevalence
  - Community Acquired
  - Hospital Acquired
  - Unit Acquired
- Psychiatric Physical/Sexual Assault Rate
- Restraint Prevalence★

- RN Education/Certification
- RN Satisfaction Survey Options
  - Job Satisfaction Scales
  - Job Satisfaction Scales—Short Form
  - Practice Environment Scale (PES)★
- Skill Mix★: Percent of total nursing hours supplied by:
  - RN's
  - LPN/LVN's
  - UAP
  - % of total nursing hours supplied by Agency Staff

Pending Indicators for 2007

- Voluntary Nurse Turnover★
- Nosocomial Infections★
  - Urinary catheter-associated urinary tract infection (UTI)
  - Central line catheter associated blood stream infection (CABSI)
  - Ventilator-associated pneumonia (VAP)

★NQF Endorsed.

[1]Visit NDNQI's website, www.nursingquality.org for full details of all NDNQI indicators.

[2]All indicators are collected and reported quarterly except for the RN Satisfaction Options which occur annually.

[3]Comparison's reports are provided based on patient, unit type and hospital bed size, e.g. Adult Medical, hospital size 100–199.

Appendix B.
National Quality Forum Indicators

TABLE 1

National Voluntary Consensus Standards for Nursing-Sensitive Care

Framework Category	Measure	Description
Patient-centered outcome measures	1. Death among surgical inpatients with treatable serious complications (failure to rescue)	Percentage of major surgical inpatients who experience a hospital-acquired complication (i.e., sepsis, pneumonia, gastrointestinal bleeding, shock/cardiac arrest, deep vein thrombosis/pulmonary embolism) and die
	2. Pressure ulcer prevalence	Percentage of inpatients who have a hospital-acquired pressure ulcer (Stage 2 or greater)
	3. Falls prevalence★	Number of inpatient falls per inpatient days
	4. Falls with injury	Number of inpatient falls with injuries per inpatient days
	5. Restraint prevalence (vest and limb only)	Percentage of inpatients who have a vest or limb restraint
	6. Urinary catheter-associated urinary tract infection (UTI) for intensive care unit (ICU) patients★	Rate of UTI associated with use of urinary catheters for ICU patients
	7. Central line catheter-associated blood stream infection rate for ICU and high-risk nursery (HRN) patients★	Rate of blood stream infections associated with use of central line catheters for ICU and HRN patients
	8. Ventilator-associated pneumonia for ICU and HRN patients★	Rate of pneumonia associated with use of ventilators for ICU patients and HRN patients
Nursing-centered intervention measures	9. Smoking cessation counseling for acute myocardial infarction (AMI)★	Percentage of AMI inpatients with history of smoking within the past year who received smoking cessation advice or counseling during hospitalization

continued next page

TABLE 1 (cont.)
National Voluntary Consensus Standards for Nursing-Sensitive Care

Framework Category	Measure	Description
Nursing-centered intervention measures (cont.)	10. Smoking cessation counseling for heart failure (HF)★	Percentage of HF inpatients with history of smoking within the past year who received smoking cessation advice or counseling during hospitalization
	11. Smoking cessation counseling for pneumonia★	Percentage of pneumonia inpatients with history of smoking within the past year who received smoking cessation advice or counseling during hospitalization
System-centered measures	12. Skill mix (Registered Nurse [RN], Licensed Vocational/Practical Nurse [LVN/LPN], unlicensed assistive personnel [UAP], and contract)	• Percentage of RN care hours to total nursing care hours • Percentage of LVN/LPN care hours to total nursing care hours • Percentage of UAP care hours to total nursing care hours • Percentage of contract hours (RN, LVN/LPN, and UAP) to total nursing care hours
	13. Nursing care hours per patient day (RN, LVN/LPN, and UAP)	• Number of RN care hours per patient day • Number of nursing staff hours (RN, LVN/LPN, UAP) per patient day
	14. Practice Environment Scale-Nursing Work Index (PES-NWI) (composite and five subscales)	Composite score and mean presence scores for each of the following subscales derived from the PES/NWI: • Nurse participation in hospital affairs • Nursing foundations for quality of care • Nurse manager ability, leadership, and support of nurses • Staffing and resource adequacy • Collegial nurse-physician relations
	15. Voluntary turnover	Number of voluntary uncontrolled separations during the month for RNs and advanced practice nurses, LVN/LPNs, and nurse assistants/aides

★ NQF-endorsed national voluntary consensus standard for hospital care.

Source: National Quality Forum (2004). *National Consensus Standards for Nursing Sensitive Care: An initial performance measure set.* Washington, DC: National Quality Forum. Page 14.

Reproduced with permission.

Index

A

Advocate Lutheran General Hospital and use of assaults indicator, 9–18
American Nurses Association and NDQNI, 1–2
Assaults indicator, 7
    experiences using, 11–28
    facilities using, 10–12, 20–24

B

Balanced score cards (PI/QI tools), 37–38, 109–110, 155
    example of using, 127–138
See also Quality measurement and reporting; Report cards

C

Children's Hospital–Omaha and use of RN satisfaction indicator, 129–138
Christiana Care Health System and use of HAPU indicator, 79–94
Collaborative governance, 167
    See also Shared governance

D

Dashboards (PI/QI tools), 60, 160
    example of using, 9–18
Data collection (NDNQI), 2–3, 4
    assaults indicator and, 15, 16, 24
    falls indicator and, 35, 46 (figure), 48–53 passim
    HAPU indicator and, 85, 100–101, 103, 107–109, 121–123
    pain indicator and, 134, 137–138
    RN satisfaction indicator and, 147, 157
Data-driven decision making, 47, 55–63, 121

Data reporting and sharing, 59–60
    See also Quality measurement and reporting
Data sharing in quality improvement, 59–60, 95–104, 113, 167–168, 171
Decision making
    data-driven, 47, 55–63, 121
    RN satisfaction indicator and, 139, 149, 150, 168–170, 172
    shared, 21, 84
    See also Nursing councils; Shared governance
Donabedian, Avedis, healthcare quality contributions, 2

F

Fall prevention and management. *See* Falls indicator
Falls indicator, 31
    experiences using, 31–75
    facilities using, 32–35, 42–43, 56–57, 66–69

G

Good Samaritan Hospital Medical Center and use of RN satisfaction indicator, 153–162

H

High Point Regional Hospital and use of falls indicator, 31–40
Hospital acquired pressure ulcers (HAPU) indicator, 76
experiences using, 79–125
facilities using, 80–84, 96–100, 106–108, 117–121

I

Institute of Medicine (IOM) reports on healthcare quality, 3

J

Job satisfaction, 139, 145, 146–147, 149, 159 (figure), 160 (table)
    example of improvement, 163–172
    See also RN satisfaction indicator
Johnson City Medical Center and use of falls indicator, 41–54

M

Mary Greeley Medical Center and use of assaults indicator, 19–28
Mental health indicators. *See* Assaults indicator
Michael DeBakey Veterans Affairs Medical Center, 141–152
Morristown Memorial Hospital and use of HAPU indicator, 95–104

N

National Database of Nursing Quality Indicators (NDNQI), 1–4
    quality indicators (list), 173
National Quality Forum (NDF), 3
    quality indicators (list), 175–176
NDNQI RN Satisfaction Survey. *See* RN Satisfaction Survey
    NDNQI start-up considerations
    assaults indicator, 12, 24
    falls indicator, 35–36, 46–47, 59–60
    HAPU indicator, 84, 100, 108–109, 122–123
    pain management indicator, 312–133
    RN satisfaction indicator, 148, 157–158
Nightingale, Florence, healthcare statistics contributions, 2
Nurse satisfaction. *See* Job satisfaction; RN satisfaction indicator
Nursing-centered intervention quality measures (NQF's), 175–176
Nursing councils and quality improvement, 14, 47–50, 59–64, 84–85, 100–109, 121–124, 134–135, 148–149, 165, 165–171
    diagram showing, 158
    leadership councils, 36, 55–64
Nursing governance, 12–14
    See also Shared governance
Nursing quality indicators. *See* Quality indicators
Nursing-sensitive indicators, 1, 3–4

NDNQI development of, 3–4
See also Quality indicators

P

Pain Assessment/Intervention/Reassessment Cycle indicator. *See* Pain management indicator
Pain management indicator, 127
    experience using, 127–138,
    facility using, 130–134
    Palomar Pomerado Health System and use of HAPU indicator, 105–116
Patient Falls indicator. *See* Falls indicator
Patient-centered outcome quality measures (NQF's), 175
Patient outcomes improvements, 1–4
Patient Safety and Quality Initiative (ANA), 1
Pay for performance (P4P) in healthcare quality, 4
PDCA/PDSA methods and models of PI/QI, 61, 85–86, 109
    examples of applying, 24–25, 88–94, 111–115
    PDSA, 100, 133, 149
Performance improvement (PI), 36, 84, 121–122, 149, 158 (diagram), 163, 167, 171
    cycle of implementing, 108, 144
    example of system-wide, 46–54
    example of unit-based, 84–90
    methods and models (PDCA/PDSA), 24–25, 61, 85–86, 88–94, 100, 109, 111-115, 133, 149
    rapid-cycle,133
    See also PDCA/PDSA methods and models; Quality improvement
Physical/Sexual Assaults indicator. *See* Assaults indicator
Plan-Do-Check-Act (PDCA) and Plan-Do-Study-Act (PDSA). *See* PDCA/PDSA methods and models
Pressure Ulcer Prevalence indicator. *See* Hospital-acquired pressure ulcers

Q

Quality improvement (QI)
    development of, 2
    methodologies and approaches (PDCA/PDSA), 25, 85, 133, 149
    nursing-sensitive indicators and, 3
    See also Performance improvement; Quality improvement of indicators